SURGICAL
OSCES
FOR MEDICAL STUDENTS

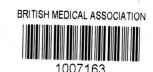

SURGICAL
OSCES

FOR MEDICAL STUDENTS

MANDA RAZ
AND LIANG LOW

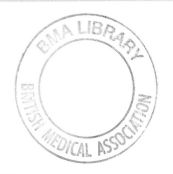

© Scion Publishing Ltd, 2019

ISBN 9781911510376

First published 2019

A CIP catalogue record for this book is available from the British Library.

Scion Publishing Limited

The Old Hayloft, Vantage Business Park, Bloxham Road, Banbury OX16 9UX, UK

www.scionpublishing.com

Important Note from the Publisher

The information contained within this book was obtained by Scion Publishing Ltd from sources believed by us to be reliable. However, while every effort has been made to ensure its accuracy, no responsibility for loss or injury whatsoever occasioned to any person acting or refraining from action as a result of information contained herein can be accepted by the authors or publishers.

Readers are reminded that medicine is a constantly evolving science and while the authors and publishers have ensured that all dosages, applications and practices are based on current indications, there may be specific practices which differ between communities. You should always follow the guidelines laid down by the manufacturers of specific products and the relevant authorities in the country in which you are practising.

Although every effort has been made to ensure that all owners of copyright material have been acknowledged in this publication, we would be pleased to acknowledge in subsequent reprints or editions any omissions brought to our attention.

Registered names, trademarks, etc. used in this book, even when not marked as such, are not to be considered unprotected by law.

Cover design by Andrew Magee Design Limited

Typeset by Medlar Publishing Solutions Pvt Ltd, India
Printed in the UK

Last digit is the print number: 10 9 8 7 6 5 4 3 2 1

Contents

List of contributors

The people named below authored a number of the stations as follows:

- Dr Emma Cole wrote stations 6, 33–35, 42 and 64
- Dr Alice Lee wrote stations 51 to 60
- Dr Peter Lioufas wrote stations 11 to 20
- Dr Kerry Liu wrote stations 31, 32 and 36–40
- Dr Fiona Pavan wrote stations 1–5 and 7–10
- Dr Emma-Leigh Rudduck wrote stations 41 and 43–50
- Dr Darius Tan wrote stations 21 to 30
- Dr Eren Tan wrote stations 61–63 and 65–68

All authors were based at Monash Medical Centre, Clayton, Victoria, Australia, at the time of writing.

Preface

The knowledge and skills required to perform well in the surgical Objective Structured Clinical Examination (OSCE) can be learnt through:

- having a clear and solid study guide
- following a step-wise approach to addressing surgical problems
- practising with colleagues.

Surgical OSCEs for Medical Students offers all the above. The book is a well-prepared written resource, outlined in a convenient structure reflecting the sequential components of patient assessment, and encourages the reader to practise with peers.

Our book presents OSCEs as physical complaints, thus maintaining true fidelity to real clinical experience. For example, patients do not seek surgical care for appendicitis, but for abdominal pain. This method will help students consolidate practical information conducive to better examination performance.

The book is prepared with the busy student in mind. Bullet points replace paragraphs, summaries substitute heavy texts, and tables supplant articles. The content has been carefully selected to achieve a balance between detail and relevancy, therefore ensuring focused and productive study time.

We wish you all the best with your surgical OSCEs.

Manda Raz (MBBS) and Liang Low (MBBS, FRACS)
Monash Health, Victoria, Australia

Acknowledgements

We would like to thank our reviewer, Dr Samuel Chee, for ensuring consistency between stations.

List of abbreviations

AAA	Abdominal aortic aneurysm	DHEA	Dehydroepiandrosterone
Ab	Antibody	DI	Diabetes insipidus
ABG	Arterial blood gas	DIP	Distal interphalangeal
ADH	Atypical ductal hyperplasia	DKA	Diabetic ketoacidosis
ADT	Androgen deprivation therapy	DM	Diabetes mellitus
AF	Atrial fibrillation	DMD	Duchenne muscular dystrophy
AFP	Alpha-fetoprotein	DRE	Digital rectal examination
ALP	Alkaline phosphatase	DRSABCD	Danger, Response, Send for help, Airway, Breathing, Circulation, Disability
AMI	Acute myocardial infarction		
ANA	Antinuclear antibody	DSA	Digital subtraction angiogram
ANCA	Antineutrophil cytoplasmic antibody	DVT	Deep vein thrombosis
AP	Anteroposterior	EBV	Epstein–Barr virus
ASIS	Anterior superior iliac spine	eGFR	Estimated glomerular filtration rate
AXR	Abdominal X-ray	EMG	Electromyography
BCC	Basal cell carcinoma	ENA	Extractable nuclear antigen
BMI	Body mass index	ERCP	Endoscopic retrograde cholangiopancreatography
BP	Blood pressure		
BPH	Benign prostatic hyperplasia	ESR	Erythrocyte sedimentation rate
BPPV	Benign paroxysmal positional vertigo	FBC	Full blood count
		FNA	Fine needle aspiration
CCB	Calcium channel blocker	FSH	Follicle-stimulating hormone
CCF	Congestive cardiac failure	GCS	Glasgow Coma Scale
CCP	Cyclic citrullinated peptide	GGT	Gamma-glutamyltransferase
CEA	Carcinoembryonic antigen	GH	Growth hormone
CK	Creatinine kinase	GI	Gastrointestinal
CMP	Calcium, magnesium, phosphate	GORD	Gastro-oesophageal reflux disease
CMV	Cytomegalovirus	Hb	Haemoglobin
COPD	Chronic obstructive pulmonary disease	hCG	Human chorionic gonadotrophin
		HDL	High-density lipoprotein
CRP	C-reactive protein	HDU	High-dependency unit
CSF	Cerebrospinal fluid	HIV	Human immunodeficiency virus
CT	Computed tomography	HL	Hodgkin's lymphoma
CVA	Cerebrovascular accident	HPV	Human papillomavirus
CXR	Chest X-ray	HR	Heart rate
CYFRA	Cytokeratin fragment	HRT	Hormone replacement therapy
DCIS	Ductal carcinoma *in situ*	HSV	Herpes simplex virus
DGP	Deamidated gliadin peptide		

ICC	Intercostal catheter	PRL	Prolactin level
ICP	Intracranial pressure	PSA	Prostate-specific antigen
IDC	Indwelling catheter	PSC	Primary sclerosing cholangitis
IGF1	Insulin-like growth factor 1	PUD	Peptic ulcer disease
IHD	Ischaemic heart disease	PVD	Peripheral vascular disease
INR	International normalised ratio	RF	Rheumatoid factor
IV	Intravenous	RIF	Right iliac fossa
LDH	Lactate dehydrogenase	ROM	Range of movement
LDL	Low-density lipoprotein	RR	Respiratory rate
LFTs	Liver function tests	RUQ	Right upper quadrant
LH	Luteinising hormone	SAAG	Serum-ascites albumin gradient
LL	Lower limb	SBP	Spontaneous bacterial peritonitis
MCP	Metacarpophalangeal	SCLC	Small cell lung cancer
MCS	Microscopy, culture and sensitivity	SCM	Sternocleidomastoid
MRCP	Magnetic resonance cholangiopancreatography	SOB	Shortness of breath
MRI	Magnetic resonance imaging	T2DM	Type 2 diabetes mellitus
MRSA	Methicillin-resistant *Staphylococcus aureus*	TACE	Transcatheter arterial chemoembolisation
NHL	Non-Hodgkin's lymphoma	TB	Tuberculosis
NKDA	No known drug allergies	TBG	Thyroxine-binding globulin
NPH	Normal pressure hydrocephalus	TFTs	Thyroid function tests
NSAID	Non-steroidal anti-inflammatory drug	TIA	Transient ischaemic attack
NSCLC	Non-small cell lung cancer	TNM	Tumour, nodes, metastasis
NSE	Neurone-specific enolase	TPO	Thyroid peroxidase
PBC	Primary biliary cirrhosis	TSH	Thyroid-stimulating hormone
PCR	Polymerase chain reaction	tTG	Tissue transglutaminase
PE	Pulmonary embolism	TTR	Transthyretin
PET	Positron emission tomography	U&Es	Urea and electrolytes
PIP	Proximal interphalangeal	UL	Upper limb
PMN	Polymorphonuclear neutrophil	US	Ultrasound
PPI	Proton pump inhibitor	UTI	Urinary tract infection
		WCC	White cell count

Station 1 **Abdominal distension**

A 65-year-old woman presents to the emergency department with abdominal pain and distension.

Tasks

1 Take a history
2 Perform a physical examination

3 Describe appropriate investigations
4 Formulate a management plan

Differential diagnoses (VIITAMINC)

Vascular:
- Portal hypertension
- Hepatic congestion
- Congestive cardiac failure
- Constrictive pericarditis
- Hepatic venous outflow obstruction
- Portal vein thrombosis

Infective:
- Spontaneous bacterial peritonitis
- Secondary bacterial peritonitis
- Tuberculous peritonitis

Inflammatory:
- Pancreatitis

Trauma

Autoimmune

Metabolic:
- Cirrhosis
- Alcoholic hepatitis

Iatrogenic

Neoplastic:
- Metastatic liver disease
- Peritoneal carcinomatosis
- Hepatocellular carcinoma
- Mesothelioma
- Other cancer – metastatic (i.e. ovarian, bowel, oesophageal, etc)

Congenital

Other:
- Nephrotic syndrome
- Lymphatic obstruction / leakage
- Hypoalbuminaemia

Before starting

Establish rapport:
- Introduce yourself
- Obtain consent to take a history and examine the patient
- Exposure: explain to the patient that you will need to do an abdominal examination

Confirm patient details:
- Name   *Jin Yong*
- Age   *65 years*
- Occupation   *Legal secretary*

History

History of presenting complaint (SOCRATES)

- **S**ite: *generalised abdominal*
- **O**nset: *gradual, constant*
- **C**haracter: *pressing, dull ache*
- **R**adiation: *nil*
- **A**ssociated symptoms: *feels bloated and swollen*
- **T**ime: *constant and worsening over 3/52*

Exacerbating / relieving: *becoming more short of breath (SOB) with enlarging abdomen*

Severity: *SOB starting to limit activities of daily living, clothes not fitting*

Take a focused history

- Cirrhosis:
  - Alcohol history: *may drink a glass of sparkling wine at social functions*
  - History of high cholesterol / obesity: *normal BMI*
  - History of intravenous drug use: *no*
  - Melaena / haematemesis: *no*
  - Skin changes:
    - Jaundice: *no*
    - Pruritus: *no*
    - Sclera colour changes: *no*
    - Easy bruising: *no*
- Cardiac failure:
  - Ischaemic heart disease (IHD) history and risk factors: *no IHD, history of type 2 diabetes mellitus (T2DM; diet-controlled)*
  - History of arrhythmia: *no*
  - Ankle / peripheral oedema: *no*
  - Smoker: *no*
- Infective:
  - Fevers / sweats / rigors: *no*
  - Sick contacts: *no*
  - Coryzal symptoms or recent viral illness: *no*
- Malignant:
  - Recent unexplained loss of weight: *3kg in 3 months*
  - Lethargy: *yes*
  - Loss of appetite: *yes*
- Other:
  - Difficulty swallowing: *no*
  - Nausea / vomiting: *mild nausea, no vomiting*
  - Bowels: *normally opens bowel daily, denies per rectal bleeding or melaena*
  - Urinary symptoms: *nil*

Past medical history and family history

- Mild anaemia, patient thinks this is due to low red meat dietary intake
- T2DM – diet-controlled

- *Hepatitis B exposure while living in China*
- *Mother has T2DM, grandmother diagnosed with bowel cancer aged 60 years*

Drug history and allergies

- *Iron supplement*
- *NKDA*

Social history

- Smoking history: *non-smoker*
- Alcohol and drug history: *social drinker, nil illicit drugs*
- *Works as a legal secretary part time*
- *Born in China, emigrated to the UK 20 years ago*
- *Home with husband, has two adult children*

Examination

General inspection (ABCD-V)

- **A**ppearance: *appears well*
- **B**ody habitus: *normal BMI*
- **C**ognition: *conscious and oriented*
- **D**evices / **D**rugs: *nil*
- **V**itals: *BP 140/90mmHg, HR 88bpm; other vitals within normal limits*

Abdomen, face and hands

- General inspection: *slightly jaundiced, obviously distended abdomen*
- Hands: *mild palmar erythema, no asterixis, normal nails, no hepatic flap*
- Face: *scleral icterus present, no mouth ulcers, normal dentition*
- Inspection (looking for peripheral stigmata of liver disease):
  - *Mild jaundice*
  - *Mildly distended abdomen*
  - *Stretch marks*
  - *No scratch marks (sign of pruritus)*
  - *No ecchymosis*
  - *Some spider naevi*
  - *No caput medusae*
- Palpation: *generalised tenderness over entire abdomen, unable to localise pain, no peritonism,*

- no guarding, no rebound or cross tenderness, no flank tenderness
- Hepatomegaly with liver extending 1cm beyond the costal margin
- No splenomegaly

- Percussion: *dull throughout and shifting dullness present*
- Hernial orifices: *small umbilical hernia, reducible*
- Digital rectal examination: *normal, no masses, no melaena, no blood*

Investigations

BBMI-O: Bedside, **B**loods, **M**icrobiology, **I**maging and **O**ther

Investigation	Rationale
Bedside	
Urinalysis via dipstick	Looking for markers of infection, haematuria or proteinuria
Blood sugar level	Insulin resistance is a complication of liver cirrhosis
Bloods	
FBC	Looking for infection, anaemia, macrocytosis and thrombocytopenia
CRP	Looking for infection
U&Es and creatinine	Looking for electrolyte imbalances and renal injury
LFTs / lipase	Liver enzymes and looking for hypoalbuminaemia (liver screen)
B$_{12}$ and iron studies	History of anaemia and part of liver screen (ferritin levels and for haemochromatosis)
Coagulation profile	Part of liver screen
Liver screen: • Hepatitis serology: A, B and C • Viral screen • CMV and EBV • Alpha-1-antitrypsin • Immunoglobulins and electrophoresis • Auto-antibody screen for autoimmune causes, i.e. PBC, PSC • AFP • Poison serum levels: if relevant exposure	Looking for causative agents to presenting illness
Microbiology – Not indicated in this case as there are clues leading to potential infection	
Imaging	
Erect AXR	If constipation or small / large bowel obstruction suspected

Investigation	Rationale
▣ Upper abdominal US	▣ First-line investigation: • Looking for the presence and quantity of ascites • Biliary system – looking for ductal dilatation, portal venous flow • Liver characterisation – nodules, lesions, smooth / irregular, inflamed (hepatitis) • Occasionally can visualise pancreas
▣ CT abdomen	To examine the liver, a standard portal venous phase CT is not always sufficient, particularly if lesions have been identified on US; can assess for metastatic disease: ▣ Triple-phase helical CT better diagnostic quality of liver lesions
▣ MRI / MRCP	More sensitive and specific than CT
Other	

▣ Abdominal paracentesis (colloquially called 'ascitic tap'	▣ To assist in diagnosing the cause and alleviating the symptoms of ascites:
	• Usually performed in the left lower quadrant, 3cm cranially and 3cm medially from the left ASIS
	• Sterile procedure
	• US guidance is suggested if patient has multiple abdominal scars or small pockets seen on US previously
	• Complications:
	  ▸ Abdominal wall haematoma
	  ▸ Haemoperitoneum
	  ▸ Bowel perforation
	  ▸ Infection

Ascitic fluid analysis

1. Visual inspection:
   • Milky – indicating the presence of chylomicrons (chylous ascites), can be caused by trauma, malignancy, cirrhosis, infection or pancreatitis
   • Cloudy – may indicate peritonitis, pancreatitis or bowel perforation
   • Bloody – malignancy or trauma
   • Straw-coloured – liver cirrhosis
2. Biochemical markers:
   • Serum-ascites albumin gradient (SAAG)
     ▸ Used to distinguish portal hypertension / hepatic congestion and other causes
     ▸ Calculation: serum albumin – ascites albumin = SAAG

SAAG >1.1mg/dL	SAAG <1.1mg/dL
Cirrhosis	Peritoneal carcinomatosis
Alcoholic hepatitis	Tuberculous peritonitis
Cardiac ascites	Pancreatic ascites
Portal vein thrombosis	Bowel obstruction
Venous obstruction	Nephrotic syndrome
	Lymphatic leak (chylous)

▓ Total protein

Transudative <30g/L protein	Exudative >30g/L protein
Cirrhosis	Venous obstruction
Cardiac ascites	Pancreatitis
Renal failure	Lymphatic obstruction
Hypoalbuminaemia	Malignancy
Nephrotic syndrome	Infection

- Amylase – investigating for pancreatic disease
- Triglycerides – for chylous ascites
- Adenosine deaminase activity (ADA) – reliable marker for tuberculosis (TB)
- Glucose – low values may indicate bacterial infection
- Lactate dehydrogenase (LDH) – high levels suggest malignancy

3. Non-biochemical markers:
   - Polymorphonuclear neutrophil (PMN) count:
     ▸ Used for patients with signs of spontaneous bacterial peritonitis (SBP)
     ▸ High PMN count can be diagnostic for SBP in the absence of other intra-abdominal sources
     ▸ Repeat PMN count after 48 hours of antibiotics can distinguish between SBP and secondary bacterial peritonitis
     ▸ Culture – for bacterial causative organism culturing
     ▸ Cytology – if malignancy suspected
   - Red cell count:
     ▸ Elevated levels may indicate malignancy
     ▸ Extreme levels indicate intra-abdominal trauma
   - White cell count and Gram stain:
     ▸ Infection, SBP, cirrhosis or TB
     ▸ Gram-positive cocci – primary peritonitis
     ▸ Gram-negative organisms – secondary peritonitis

Diagnosis

Hepatocellular carcinoma

Signs of acute liver disease with weight loss and a previous history of hepatitis B exposure should raise suspicions of hepatocellular carcinoma.

The gold standard investigation to confirm hepatocellular carcinoma is MRI:
▓ *Triple-phase CT*
▓ *MRI*
▓ *Biopsy not always needed as radiological findings may be sufficient*

Discussion

It is a primary liver cancer, more common in people with cirrhosis (i.e. due to chronic liver inflammation).

It is more common in Asian countries.

Risk factors:
▓ Viral hepatitis (hepatitis B or C)
▓ Exposure to toxins
▓ Alcoholic liver cirrhosis
▓ T2DM
▓ Haemochromatosis
▓ Alpha-1 antitrypsin deficiency

Management

▓ Four possible approaches: to cure, bridging (while waiting for liver transplant), downstaging (tumour burden reduction) or palliative (symptom management)

- Symptomatic / palliative:
  - Diet: sodium restriction
  - Fluid restriction: aim for less than 2L per day
  - Diuretics: furosemide ± spironolactone
  - Therapeutic paracentesis (ascitic tap)
- Surgical resection:
  - Hemihepatectomy
  - Requiring extensive preoperative planning to ensure enough functional liver remaining after resection
  - Higher risk of morbidity and mortality with liver cirrhosis
- Liver transplant
- Ablation:
  - Radiofrequency ablation:
    - High-frequency radio waves to destroy tumours with local heat
    - Electrodes inserted into the mass via US laparoscopic or open surgical guidance
    - Can be repeated multiple times
  - Cryoablation
    - Destroying tumours with cold temperatures
    - Probe inserted into the tumour and liquid nitrogen injected
- Arterial catheter-based treatment:
  - Transcatheter arterial chemoembolisation (TACE):
    - For unresectable tumours
    - Medication cocktail of chemotherapy and embolic agents are injected into the right or left hepatic artery via the femoral artery
    - Aim is to restrict blood flow to the tumour while also delivering targeted chemotherapy agents
    - Slows tumour progression
  - Selective internal radiation therapy (SIRT):
    - Similar to TACE; however, radiotherapy is delivered to the tumour
    - Non-curative, slows disease progression

Other differential diagnoses

- Liver cirrhosis

Station 2 **Abdominal mass**

A 40-year-old woman presents to the emergency department with 1 week of right iliac fossa (RIF) abdominal pain and new swelling.

Tasks

1 Take a history
2 Perform a targeted examination
3 Describe appropriate investigations
4 Formulate a management plan

Differential diagnoses (VIITAMINC)

Vascular:
- Ruptured abdominal aortic aneurysm (AAA)

Infective:
- Appendicitis
- Diverticulitis
- Abscess

Inflammatory:
- Inflammatory bowel disease
- Endometriosis

Traumatic:
- Trauma

Autoimmune

Metabolic

Iatrogenic

Neoplastic:
- Malignancy – ovarian, bowel, uterine, peritoneal

Congenital

Other:
- Small bowel obstruction
- Large bowel obstruction / volvulus
- Incarcerated hernia
- Constipation
- Ovarian torsion / cyst
- Ectopic pregnancy
- Ingested foreign body

Before starting

Establish rapport:
- Introduce yourself
- Obtain consent to take a history and examine the patient
- Exposure: explain to the patient that, if indicated, a digital rectal examination (DRE) may be required and consider the need for a chaperone

Confirm patient details:
- Name — *Sally Smith*
- Age — *40*
- Occupation — *School teacher*

History

History of presenting complaint (SOCRATES)
- **S**ite: *localised to right iliac fossa but initially was generalised*
- **O**nset: *gradual increase over the past week*
- **C**haracter: *sharp, stabbing*
- **R**adiation: *nil*
- **A**ssociated symptoms: *malaise, feels feverish, one episode of vomit and diarrhoea 3 days ago*
- **T**ime: *constant*
- **E**xacerbating / relieving: *exacerbated by walking / moving, not affected by food*
- **S**everity: *has gradually increased to 8/10*

Take a focused history

- Oral / oesophagus:
  - Vomiting: *one bilious vomit today, no haematemesis, no coffee ground vomitus*
  - Swallowing difficulties: *no*
  - Diet / appetite: *usually good, loss of appetite over the past 5 days*
- Stomach:
  - Reflux symptoms: *no*
  - If suspected, risk factors for peptic ulcer disease (PUD): *no*
- Bowels:
  - Bowels last opened: *3 days ago*
  - Bowel action history: *usually regular brown, no per rectal bleeding or melaena*
  - Colour / consistency of bowel actions: *mild diarrhoea 3 days ago, no blood / mucus*
- Genitourinary system:
  - Dysuria, haematuria or urinary frequency: *no*
  - Possibly pregnant / sexual history: *on oral contraceptive pill, no barrier contraception, sexually active with husband, has regular periods*
  - Back pain: *no*
- Systemic (**SWIM**):
  - **S**kin: *no recent jaundice / stretch marks / itch / pallor*
  - **W**eight: *no recent unexplained loss of weight or fatigue*
  - **I**nfective:
    - Fevers / sweats / rigors: *feverish, rigors overnight, diaphoretic*
    - Sick contacts: *no*
    - Coryzal symptoms or recent viral illness: *no*
    - Recent overseas travel: *no*
  - **M**usculoskeletal:
    - Joint pain: *no*
    - History of trauma: *no*

Past medical history and family history

- *Uterine fibroids*
- *Hypertension*
- *Nil significant family history*

Drug history and allergies

- *Oral contraceptive pill*
- *NKDA*

Social history

- Smoking history: *recently quit smoking*
- Alcohol and drugs history: *social drinker, no illicit drugs*
- *Full-time school teacher, home with partner and two children*

Examination

General inspection (ABCD-V)

- **A**ppearance: *patient looks diaphoretic, fatigued and unwell*
- **B**ody habitus: *normal BMI*
- **C**ognition: *conscious and oriented*
- **D**evices / **D**rugs: *nil*
- **V**itals: *BP 130/85mmHg, HR 60bpm, temperature 38.1°C; other vitals within normal limits*

Abdomen

- Exposure: *lying supine on a completely flattened bed, exposure from xiphisternum to mons pubis*
- Inspection: *no skin changes, obvious small swelling in RIF, not distended*
- Palpation: *tenderness over RIF with involuntary guarding, rebound and cross tenderness, no generalised peritonism, palpable tender non-pulsatile mass in RIF, no flank tenderness; Rovsing's sign positive; no hernial orifices*
- Percussion: *tenderness in RIF, normal percussion note*
- DRE: *normal*

Investigations

BBMI: Bedside, **B**loods, **M**icrobiology and **I**maging

Investigation	Rationale
Bedside	
Urinalysis via dipstick	Looking for markers of infection or haematuria
Urinary pregnancy test	Looking to confirm pregnancy
Blood sugar level	Looking to confirm diagnosis of diabetes mellitus
Bloods	
FBC	Looking for infection and anaemia
U&Es and creatinine	Looking for electrolyte imbalances and renal injury
CRP / ESR	Looking for raised markers as a sign of infection
LFTs / lipase	As part of an abdominal screen
Formal beta-hCG	Formally diagnoses pregnancy and indicates gestation
Tumour markers: Ca125, CEA, Ca19-9 and AFP	Not done acutely; if malignancy found can be used to monitor cancer
Microbiology	
	Not indicated in this case as there are clues leading to potential infection
Imaging	
Erect CXR	If suspected visceral perforation, looking for free gas under the diaphragm
Erect AXR	If constipation or small / large bowel obstruction suspected, can sometimes see a foreign body
Abdominal US	To examine gynaecological organs and can occasionally visualise the appendix or look for secondary signs of appendicitis (e.g. free fluid, surrounding inflammation)
CT abdomen / pelvis	Useful for characterising the mass, identifying location and management planning: • Rim-enhancing abscess • Phlegmon / inflammatory • Malignant ± lymphadenopathy or distant metastases • Amenable to biopsy or percutaneous drainage

Diagnosis

Appendicitis with phlegmon

RIF tenderness, guarding, rebound and cross tenderness and Rovsing's sign are highly indicative of appendicitis. A palpable tender mass raises the suspicion of a phlegmon.

The gold standard investigation to confirm appendicitis and phlegmon is CT abdomen/pelvis.

Pathophysiology

- Obstruction due to one of the following:
  - Usual cause is a small fragment of faecal matter (faecolith) causing obstruction
  - Tumour requiring further management e.g. carcinoid tumour
    - Most common malignant tumour of the appendix
    - Type of neuroendocrine tumour arising from enterochromaffin cells
    - Common in the small intestine, rectum and stomach
    - Treatment: surgical resection if the tumour has not metastasised or if not curable, octreotide can help to prolong survival; chemotherapy has little benefit
  - Worms (*Enterobius vermicularis*) (very rare):
    - The presence of 'pinworm' in the appendix can mimic symptoms of appendicitis, though infection with pinworm is usually asymptomatic
      - Other symptoms of pruritus ani or eosinophilia in the blood can provide a higher suspicion to an alternative diagnosis such as pinworm
  - Gallstone (very rare)
- Obstruction causes continued secretion of mucinous fluid in the appendix causing increased intraluminal pressure
- Pressure leading to collapse of the draining veins and ischaemic injury
- Ischaemic conditions favourable to bacterial proliferation with further oedema and exudate
- Inflammatory process worsens, causing abscess formation and ulceration
- Then ulcerative gangrenous necrosis, which can result in perforation

Management

Acute appendicitis

- IV antibiotics
- Laparoscopic appendicectomy ± open appendicectomy:
  - Uncomplicated – usually return home the following day
  - Gangrenous – 24–48h IV antibiotics post resection
  - Distal perforation – 48h IV antibiotics post resection
  - Proximal perforation – appendicectomy ± caecectomy with period thereafter of IV antibiotics
  - Intraoperative discovery of dense inflammation (phlegmon) with unresectable appendix – 5 days of IV antibiotics and interval appendicectomy 6–8 weeks thereafter
  - Appendicitis with lesion – right hemicolectomy

Acute appendicitis with phlegmon

- IV antibiotics for 7 days
- Colonoscopy looking for lesion/polyp
- Interval appendicectomy if colonoscopy normal

Appendicitis with contained perforation

- IV antibiotics
- CT-guided drainage of abscess
- Interval appendicectomy if remains well; if unstable, may require more urgent appendicectomy

Perforated appendicitis with peritonitis

- IV antibiotics
- Laparoscopic washout and appendicectomy ± caecectomy

Other differential diagnoses

- Ovarian cyst
- Ectopic pregnancy

Station 3 **Abdominal pain**

A 20-year-old woman presents to the emergency department with recurrent abdominal pain.

Tasks

1 Take a history
2 Perform a targeted examination

3 Describe appropriate investigations
4 Formulate a management plan

Differential diagnoses (VIITAMINC)

Vascular:
- Ischaemic bowel
- Ruptured abdominal aortic aneurysm (AAA)
- Ischaemic colitis
- Splenic infarct

Infective:
- Appendicitis
- Cholecystitis / ascending cholangitis
- Pancreatitis
- Infective colitis
- Diverticulitis
- Urinary tract infection / pyelonephritis
- Glandular fever

Inflammatory:
- Epiploic appendicitis
- Endometriosis
- Gastritis / peptic ulcer disease
- Mesenteric adenitis

Traumatic:
- Trauma

Autoimmune:
- Pancreatitis
- Inflammatory bowel disease

Metabolic:
- Diabetic ketoacidosis (DKA)

Iatrogenic

Neoplastic:
- Malignancy

Congenital

Other:
- Ectopic pregnancy
- Hollow viscous perforation
- Small bowel obstruction
- Large bowel obstruction / volvulus
- Ingested foreign body
- Incarcerated hernia
- Constipation
- Cholelithiasis / choledocholithiasis
- Ovarian torsion / abscess / ruptured cyst
- Renal colic

Before starting

Establish rapport:
- Introduce yourself
- Obtain consent to take a history and examine the patient

- Exposure: explain to the patient that you will need to do a digital rectal examination (DRE) and consider need for chaperone

Confirm patient details:
- Name — *Emily Brown*
- Age — *20 years*
- Occupation — *Student / hospitality*

History

History of presenting complaint (SOCRATES)

- **S**ite: *pain in central abdomen radiating to right iliac fossa*
- **O**nset: *gradual, intermittent*
- **C**haracter: *at times sharp, but mostly dull ache*
- **R**adiation: *none*
- **A**ssociated symptoms: *today vomiting, malaise, feels feverish*
- **T**ime: *lasts for periods during the day for hours, first started 1 month ago*
- **E**xacerbating / relieving: *exacerbated by walking / moving, not affected by food*
- **S**everity: *limiting day-to-day activities*

Take a focused history

- Oral / oesophagus:
  - Vomiting: *three bilious vomits today, no blood, no haematemesis*
  - Swallowing difficulties: *no*
  - Diet / appetite: *usually good, loss of appetite over the past 4 days*
- Stomach:
  - Reflux symptoms: *no*
  - If suspected, any risk factors for peptic ulcer disease (PUD): *no*
- Bowels:
  - Bowels last opened: *today, three motions*
  - Bowel action history: *usually alternates between diarrhoea and constipation*
  - Colour / consistency of bowel actions: *brown, occasional streaks of blood on toilet paper, occasional mucus, mild diarrhoea past 3 days*
- Genitourinary system:
  - Dysuria, haematuria or urinary frequency: *no*
  - Possibly pregnant / sexual history: *always uses protection, has not been sexually active in 6 months, has regular periods*
  - Back pain: *no*
- Systemic (**SWIM**):
  - **S**kin: *no jaundice / stretch marks / itch; others have commented on her being paler than usual; cracking and redness in both corners of the mouth and mouth ulcers*
  - **W**eight: *recent unexplained loss of 3kg in 3 months; associated fatigue*

- **I**nfective:
  - Fevers / sweats / rigors: *no*
  - Sick contacts: *no*
  - Coryzal symptoms or recent viral illness: *no*
  - Recent overseas travel: *no*
- **M**usculoskeletal:
  - Joint pain: *occasionally has sore knees and stiff fingers*
  - History of trauma: *no*

Past medical history and family history

- *Mild anaemia, likely from a low red meat dietary intake*
- *Mother has type 1 diabetes mellitus, grandmother has Crohn's disease*

Drug history and allergies

- *Oral contraceptive pill*
- *NKDA*
- *Recent course oral antibiotics for an ear infection*

Social history

- Smoking history: *recently quit*
- Alcohol and drugs history: *social drinker, no illicit drugs*
- Accommodation: *at home with family*
- Occupation: *studying architecture, works part-time in a café*

Examination

General inspection (ABCD-V)

- **A**ppearance: *patient looks pale, fatigued and unwell*
- **B**ody habitus: *normal, BMI 22*
- **C**ognition: *conscious and oriented*
- **D**evices / **D**rugs: *nil*
- **V**itals: *BP 110/65mmHg, HR 58bpm and regular; other vitals within normal limits; afebrile*

Abdomen

- Exposure: *lying supine on a completely flattened bed, exposure from xiphisternum to mons pubis*
- Inspection: *no skin changes or surgical scars, no obvious swellings*
- Palpation: *generalised tenderness over umbilicus and right iliac fossa (RIF), no rigidity / guarding / peritonism, no rebound*

or cross tenderness, no palpable masses,
no organomegaly, no hernial orifices
- Percussion: *no percussive tenderness*
- Rovsing's sign: *negative*

- Auscultation: *bowel sounds audible*
- DRE: *small perianal fissure at 12 o'clock, normal brown faeces, no mass*

Investigations

BBMI-O: Bedside, **B**loods, **M**icrobiology, **I**maging and **O**ther

Investigation	Rationale
Bedside	
Urinalysis via dipstick	Looking for markers of infection or haematuria
Urinary pregnancy test	Looking for pregnancy
Blood sugar level	Looking for diabetes
Bloods	
FBC	Looking for infection and anaemia
CRP	Looking for infection
U&Es and creatinine	Looking for electrolyte imbalances and renal injury
LFTs / lipase	Part of abdominal pain screen
Formal beta-hCG	Confirmation of pregnancy
B_{12} and iron studies	Given chronicity and history of mild anaemia
Microbiology	
Faecal analysis	Macroscopically looking for blood or mucus and colour MCS: if infection suspected Ova / cysts / parasites Calprotectin level: marker of inflammatory bowel disease
Imaging	
Erect CXR	If suspected visceral perforation, looking for free gas under the diaphragm
Erect AXR	If constipation or small / large bowel obstruction suspected, can sometimes see a foreign body
Abdominal US	Upper abdominal: to examine biliary system and occasionally can visualise pancreas; lower abdominal: to examine appendix and gynaecological organs; renal tract: if renal colic suspected
Barium swallow / gastrograffin follow through	Looking for skip lesions or luminal narrowing

Investigation	Rationale
CT abdomen / pelvis	In a young female patient the radiation risk of a CT scan should be weighed with the possible diagnostic benefit; this is not always the next investigation in patients of this demographic; however, it may be useful in the older population to evaluate other common causes of abdominal pain including malignancy
Other – in individuals where a diagnosis has not yet been made	
Diagnostic laparoscopy	Can be diagnostic and therapeutic; often done if the patient has suspected appendicitis; not uncommon to reveal other causes such as: • Ovarian pathology • Retrograde menstruation • Mesenteric adenitis • Epiploic appendicitis • Meckel's diverticulum • Bowel tumour / peritoneal disease
Colonoscopy / gastroscopy	May be negative or elicit unclear results; can aid in the diagnosis of: • Inflammatory bowel disease with views to the terminal ileum • Polyps / cancer • PUD / gastritis
Pill cam	To evaluate the small bowel; unable to obtain biopsies

Diagnosis

Crohn's disease

A history of alternating bowel habits, unexplained weight loss, arthralgia, mouth ulcers, angular stomatitis, a family history of inflammatory bowel disease and a relatively benign examination apart from an anal fissure is highly suggestive of inflammatory bowel disease. Crohn's disease tends to affect the entire alimentary tract, and so mouth ulcers and angular stomatitis are more common in Crohn's as compared with ulcerative colitis.

The gold standard investigation to confirm Crohn's disease is a colonoscopy with tissue biopsy.

Discussion

What is Crohn's disease?

- Chronic inflammatory autoimmune condition of the digestive tract – can affect anywhere from the mouth to the anus
- It is a type of inflammatory bowel disease that affects 0.32% of the developed population
- Common symptoms include abdominal pain, bloody or mucous diarrhoea, fever and weight loss; signs and symptoms are not limited to the gastrointestinal tract
- The cause is unknown; however, genetically susceptible individuals may develop Crohn's due to a combination of immune, environmental and bacterial factors

- Those with the disease are at higher risk of bowel cancer
- There is no cure; treatment options are aimed at symptom minimisation and complication management
- Symptoms often follow a flare and resolving pattern, with patients often having had years of symptoms before diagnosis

Other examination findings and associated conditions of Crohn's disease:
- DRE:
  - red inflamed anus (proctitis) ± tenderness
  - perianal inflammation: abscesses, haemorrhoids, anal fissures / fistulae, skin tags
- Digit clubbing
- Uveitis / iritis
- Arthropathy
- Erythema nodosum:
  - Raised tender nodules on the shins
- Pyoderma gangrenosum:
  - Painful ulcerating nodules / ulcers
- Other manifestations of malnutrition
- Mouth ulcers and stomatitis
- Seronegative spondyloarthropathy:
  - Arthritis
  - Sacroiliitis
  - Ankylosing spondylitis
- Osteoporosis
- Depression

Risk factors:
- Tobacco smoking
- Living near an industrial zone

Investigation findings of Crohn's disease:
- CT:
  - Useful for looking for intra-abdominal abscesses, small bowel obstructions or fistulae
- Barium swallow / follow through:
  - To examine the small intestine not accessible to endoscopy
  - Can demonstrate inflammation and narrowing suggestive of strictures – string of Kantor, fistulae, rose thorn ulcers
- Colonoscopy / sigmoidoscopy:
  - Views to terminal ileum

- Macroscopic cobblestone-like appearance of ulcers and scarring
- Non-caseating crypt granulomas containing multinucleated giant cells
- MRI:
  - Sensitive enough to detect ulceration and inflammation
- Biopsy:
  - Neutrophil infiltrations in crypts and mucosal inflammation
  - Involves the whole bowel wall (transmural inflammation)
  - Villi blunting, atypical branching of crypts
  - Metaplasia – Paneth cell metaplasia

Management

Aimed at treating the acute symptoms and then maintaining remission.

Lifestyle

- Avoiding triggers (milk, polyunsaturated fats, stress)
- Eating smaller amounts more often
- Smoking cessation
- Higher-fibre diet to prevent; however, low-fibre during flares
- Oral caloric supplements

Medical

- Antibiotics and corticosteroids in acute flare
- Immunomodulators (e.g. azathioprine, methotrexate, infliximab)
- Hydrocortisone in severe attacks
- Total parenteral nutrition (TPN) in cases of severe malnourishment
- Electrolyte replacement

Surgical

- Not curative, often needed if no relief after medical therapy
- Can be used to resect areas of partial or full intestinal blockage or resection / debridement of fistulae or abscesses
- Postsurgical recurrence is fairly common
- Perforation most commonly occurs at the terminal ileum which may then be resected

Complications associated with Crohn's disease

- Bowel obstruction secondary to fibrosis or stricture
- Perforation
- Fistulae:
  - Colovesical – pneumaturia, recurrent urinary tract infections
  - Colovaginal – faecal vaginal discharge
  - Enterocutaneous – skin abscess ± faecal discharge
- Colorectal carcinoma / lymphoma
- Malabsorption / malnutrition:
  - B_{12} deficiency – especially after ileal resection
  - Iron-deficiency anaemia – due to chronic blood loss and reduced duodenal absorption
- Bile salt malabsorption (with disease affecting the ileum) causing cholesterol gallstones and kidney stones

Other differential diagnoses

- Ulcerative colitis
- Colitis / gastrointestinal infection:
  - *Clostridium difficile*, shigella, salmonella
  - *Giardia* spp.
  - Yersinia ileitis
  - Amoebic dysentery
- Irritable bowel disease
- Coeliac disease
- Colorectal cancer
- Rare:
  - NSAID drug enteropathy
  - Intestinal tuberculosis

Crohn's disease versus ulcerative colitis

	Crohn's disease	Ulcerative colitis
Tenesmus	Uncommon	Common
Fistulae	Common	Rare
Stenosis	Common	Rare
Faeces	Porridge-like Steatorrhoea Mild bleeding	Mucous Bloody
Primary sclerosing cholangitis	Less common	More common
Perianal disease	Common	Less common
Terminal ileum	Commonly affected	Rarely affected
Colon involvement	Usually	Always
Rectum involvement	Rarely	Usually
Endoscopy	Cobblestone appearance Snake-like ulcers	Continuous ulcers
Inflammation	Transmural	Shallow mucosal
Surgery	Often returns following resection of affected zones	Curative with colonic resection
Colon cancer	Small risk	High risk

Station 4 **Acute confusion**

A 78-year-old woman presents to the emergency department with her family who have found her to be increasingly confused over the past 3 days.

Tasks

1 Take a history
2 Perform a targeted examination
3 Describe appropriate investigations

4 Interpret these blood results
5 Formulate a management plan

Differential diagnoses

Red flags (4Hs and 4Ts):

- **H**ypotension
- **H**ypoxia
- **H**ypoglycaemia / electrolyte derangement
- **H**ypothermia / hyperthermia
- **T**ension pneumothorax
- **T**ablets / toxins
- **T**amponade
- **T**hrombosis / embolism (myocardial infarction or pulmonary embolism (PE))

(VIITAMINC)

Vascular:
- Thrombosis / embolism (acute myocardial infarction (AMI) or PE)
- Congestive cardiac failure
- Stroke / transient ischaemic attack (TIA)
- Intracranial haemorrhage
- Anaemia

Infective:
- Pneumonia
- Urinary tract infection
- Gastroenteritis
- Influenza
- Meningitis

Inflammatory

Trauma:
- Head injury / contusion

Autoimmune

Metabolic:
- Hepatic encephalopathy
- Renal impairment
- Thyroid dysfunction
- Electrolyte disturbance

Iatrogenic

Neoplastic:
- Malignancy + paraneoplastic syndromes

Congenital:
- Epilepsy / seizures

Other:
- Psychosis
- Dementia
- Pain
- Nutrition
- Sleeplessness
- Environmental change

Before starting

Establish rapport:
- Introduce yourself
- Obtain consent to take a history and examine the patient:

- In a patient acutely confused, they may not be able to consent
- For a consent to be valid it must fulfil the following (**VIC**):
  - **V**oluntary – without pressure or coercion

- ▸ **I**nformed – full disclosure of the nature of the procedure / examination including the benefits and risks
- ▸ **C**apacity – the patient must be able to comprehend the information provided
- Exposure: explain what is likely to occur, including the need for appropriate exposure during the examination

Confirm patient details:
- Name   *Sue Short*
- Age   *78 years*
- Occupation   *Retired*

History

Take a history from the patient themselves – as best as possible:
- Aids in determining current mental state
- Assess Glasgow Coma Score (GCS) and orientation to person / place / time; useful as a baseline
- What are they seeing / hearing / feeling?
- Gentle reorientation if indicated

Collateral history

Ask about the confusion:
- Duration: *5 days*
- Onset: *gradual at first, very noticeable now*
- What has changed: *usually patient shops and cooks for herself, now forgetful of where her bedroom is, found wandering outside*
- First presentation: *yes*

Focused history

- Infective symptoms:
  - Fevers / sweats / rigors: *no*
  - Vomiting / diarrhoea: *yes, 1 week ago everyone had food poisoning after a family birthday*
  - Cough, coryzal symptoms: *no*
  - Open wounds / injuries: *no*
- Skin changes: *paler than usual, no jaundice / itch*
- Functional issues:
  - Recent fall: *no*
  - Issues with sleep or recent environmental change: *no*
  - Pain: *no*
  - Behavioural change: *no*
- Cardiac:
  - Palpitations: *no*
  - Dyspnoea: *no*
  - Chest pain: *no*
- Malignancy:
  - Weight loss or change in appetite: *old food still in a very full fridge*
  - Melaena / per rectal bleeding: *no*
  - Haemoptysis / haematemesis: *no*
- Neurological:
  - Seizure activity: *no*
  - Paralysis or paraesthesia: *no*
  - Swallowing difficulties / dysphagia: *no*
  - Changes to speech / aphasia: *no*
  - Head strike / injury: *no*
  - Headaches / change in vision: *no*

Past medical history and family history

- *Hypertension*
- *Atrial fibrillation*
- *Varicose veins*
- *Osteoporosis*
- *Nil significant family history*

Drug history and allergies

- *Furosemide*
- *Warfarin*
- *Ramipril*

Social history

- Smoking history: *recently quit smoking, previously heavy smoker*

- Alcohol and drugs history: *nil alcohol, no illicit drugs*
- Lives home alone in retirement village
- Usually independent with activities of daily living, home help with house cleaning fortnightly
- Nil gait aids

Examination

General inspection (ABCD-V):

- **A**ppearance: *patient looks fatigued and unwell with dry lips*
- **B**ody habitus: *normal, BMI 23*
- **C**ognition: *conscious, sleepy and disoriented*
- **D**evices / **D**rugs: *nil*
- **V**itals: *BP 90/50mmHg, HR 105bpm, RR 18 breaths per minute; oxygen saturation at 97% on room air; afebrile*

Fluid assessment

- General inspection:
  - Short of breath / respiratory distress: *no*
  - Visible oedema (fluid overload): *mild pitting oedema to ankles bilaterally*
  - Skin colour: *pale*
  - Other devices (stoma bags, drain tubes, IV drips): *no*
  - Wounds: *no*
- Vital signs: *as above*
- Charts / data (if available, otherwise request as part of management):
  - Fluid balance chart
  - Drain tube chart
  - Weight
  - Stool chart
  - Medications and IV fluids chart

- Hands:
  - Capillary refill: *<2 seconds*
  - Radial pulse – character and rate: *strong, regular 105bpm*
  - Peripheral stigmata of liver or renal disease: *no*
- Arms:
  - Peripheral temperature: *36.9°C*
  - Postural blood pressure: *85/50mmHg*
- Face:
  - Eyes – sunken or periorbital oedema: *normal*
  - Mucous membranes: *moist*
  - Conjunctiva – jaundice or anaemia: *no*
- Neck:
  - Jugular venous pressure visualisation: *+2cm from sterna angle*
  - Use of accessory respiratory muscles: *no*
- Torso:
  - Chest auscultation of lungs and heart sounds: *dual heart sounds no murmurs (DHSNM), clear lung fields*
  - Sternal capillary refill: *<2 seconds*
  - Sacral oedema: *no*
  - Shifting dullness of ascites: *no*
- Legs:
  - Peripheral oedema and to what level: *mild pitting oedema to ankles bilaterally*
  - Capillary refill: *<2 seconds*

Investigations

BBMI-O: Bedside, **B**loods, **M**icrobiology, **I**maging and **O**ther

Investigation	Rationale
Bedside	
Urinalysis via dipstick	Looking for markers of infection or haematuria
Blood sugar level	Looking for diabetes mellitus
Bloods	
FBC	Looking for infection and anaemia
CRP	Looking for infection
U&Es and creatinine	Looking for electrolyte imbalances and renal injury, especially sodium, potassium, bicarbonate and chloride, in the setting of diarrhoea and vomiting
LFTs / lipase	Liver failure or pancreatitis as the cause of vomiting
INR	Given patient is warfarinised; may be subtherapeutic if not taking medications or supratherapeutic in the setting of dehydration or sepsis
TFTs	Confusion in hypothyroid states
Blood cultures	If sepsis suspected; elderly patients may not mount a systemic response of fevers so important to consider cold sepsis in the confused elderly patient
Microbiology	
	Not indicated in this case, as there are clues leading to potential infection
Imaging	
CXR (PA and lateral views)	As part of septic screen for possible pneumonia
CT brain	Looking for stroke, intracranial bleed, malignancy / space-occupying lesion
Other	
EEG	Looking for seizure activity as a cause for confusion

Blood test results

U&Es and creatinine:
- Sodium: *119mmol/L (135–145mmol/L)*
- Potassium: *4.8mmol/L (3.5–5.0mmol/L)*
- Chloride: *99mmol/L (95–110mmol/L)*

- Bicarbonate: *26mmol/L (22–32mmol/L)*
- Urea: *6.4 mmol/L (2.8–7.2mmol/L)*
- Creatinine: *105μmol/L (60–110μmol/L)*

Estimated glomerular filtration rate (eGFR): *>90mL/min (>90mL/min)*

Diagnosis

Hyponatraemia secondary to hypovolaemia

A history of increased fluid losses (food poisoning) followed by prolonged decreased oral intake with symptoms of confusion is suggestive.

The gold standard investigation to confirm hyponatraemia from hypovolaemia is urine sodium.

Urine sodium in hypovolaemia:
- Pre-renal: urinary sodium <20mmol/L:
  - Fluid loss: sweating / vomiting / diarrhoea along with continued water intake:
    - Associated alkalosis with upper gastrointestinal (GI) and skin losses
    - Associated acidosis with lower GI losses
  - Third space losses: pancreatitis, burns, bowel obstruction
- Renal: urinary sodium >20mmol/L:
  - Diuretics (i.e. thiazides, osmotic)
  - Renal failure
  - Addison's disease
  - Syndrome of inappropriate antidiuretic hormone secretion (SIADH)

Symptoms:
Severity is associated with the rapidity of concentration loss
- Mild hyponatraemia: >125mmol/L – asymptomatic
- Moderate hyponatraemia: 115–125mmol/L – lethargy, confusion, anorexia, nausea / vomiting
- Severe hyponatraemia: <115mmol/L – muscle cramps / weakness, convulsions, coma

Management

- Depends on the pathology, in this case the patient was found to be significantly hyponatraemic and hypovolaemic due to diarrhoea and vomiting
- Short term:
  - Reorient the patient where appropriate
  - Avoid triggers such as pain or frequent room / ward changes
  - Avoid medications known to precipitate / exacerbate delirium
  - Supportive environment factors and falls assessment
- Medical
  - IV rehydration: fluid resuscitation to combat the hypovolaemic state
  - Correction, via boluses of hypertonic saline:
    - Acute severe hyponatraemia: aim for 1–2mEq/hour correction

- Chronic severe hyponatraemia: aim for 0.5–1mEq/hour correction
- Beware of rapid overcorrection, this can cause central pontine myelinolysis; causes paralysis, dysphagia, diplopia and reduced consciousness
- Do not exceed 10mmol/L in the first 24 hours
- Anti-emetic: if ongoing vomiting / nausea

Other differential diagnoses

- Dementia
- Delirium

Station 5 **Anal pain**

A 30-year-old woman presents to the emergency department with 2 days of perianal pain.

Tasks

1 Take a history
2 Perform a targeted examination

3 Describe appropriate investigations
4 Formulate a management plan

Differential diagnoses (VIITAMINC)

- **V**ascular

- **I**nfective:
  - Perianal/ischiorectal abscess
  - Proctitis
  - Perineal abscess
  - Pelvic inflammatory disease

- **I**nflammatory:
  - Pruritus ani
  - Haemorrhoids
  - Inflammatory bowel disease
  - Perianal fistula and fissure
  - Rectal ulcer
  - Coccydynia

- **T**rauma:
  - Trauma

- **A**utoimmune

- **M**etabolic

- **I**atrogenic

- **N**eoplastic:
  - Anal cancer
  - Rectal cancer
  - Pelvic cancer

- **C**ongenital

- Other:
  - Proctalgia fugax
  - Levator ani syndrome
  - Trauma
  - Foreign body
  - Endometriosis
  - Constipation

Before starting

Establish rapport:
- Introduce yourself
- Consent to take a history and examine the patient
- Exposure: explain to the patient that you will need to do a rectal examination and consider need for chaperone

Confirm patient details:
- Name   *Tess Wools*
- Age   *30 years*
- Occupation   *Personal trainer*

History

History of presenting complaint (SOCRATES)

- **S**ite: *perianal/anus pain*
- **O**nset: *gradual*
- **C**haracter: *sharp, stabbing*
- **R**adiation: *nil*
- **A**ssociated symptoms: *swelling in area*
- **T**ime: *2 days, gradually increasing, constant*
- **E**xacerbating/relieving: *exacerbated by sitting down on buttocks and with bowel actions, some relief with standing*
- **S**everity: *limiting day-to-day activities*

Take a focused history

- Perianal discharge: *no pus or mucus*
- Perianal itching: *yes, occasionally*
- Change in stool colour / PR bleeding: *small amount of blood on wiping, not mixed in with faeces, otherwise faeces brown, no melaena*
- Changes to bowel habits: *bowels usually opened daily; however, has been more constipated during pregnancy*
- History of vaginal discharge or history of sexually-transmitted infections: *no*
- History of dysuria or urinary frequency: *urinary frequency but no dysuria*
- History of anal trauma or intercourse: *no*
- Recent unexplained loss of weight: *no*
- History of systemic symptoms: *no fevers, sweats or rigors*

Past medical history and family history

- G2P1: *currently 35 weeks pregnant, uncomplicated pregnancy*
- *Varicose veins*
- *No family history of bowel cancer or irritable bowel disease*

Drug history and allergies

- *NKDA*
- *Fish oil*
- *Taking regular paracetamol for pain relief*

Social history

- Smoking history: *non-smoker*
- Alcohol and drugs history: *non-drinker, nil illicit drugs*
- *Personal trainer*
- *Currently on maternity leave*

Examination

General inspection (ABCD-V)

- **A**ppearance: *patient is in pain, lying on side and unwilling to sit up*
- **B**ody habitus: *gravid, high BMI*
- **C**ognition: *conscious and oriented*
- **D**evices / **D**rugs: *ice pack at the end of the bed*
- **V**itals: *within normal limits, afebrile*

Abdomen

- Inspection: *no surgical scars; abdominal distension with signs of pregnancy*
- Palpation: *no abdominal pain or palpable faeces, uterus palpated to epigastrium*
- Percussion: *no percussion tenderness*
- Auscultation: *normal bowel sounds present*

Anus

- Positioning: *lying left lateral*
- Inspection: *1cm swelling at 3 o'clock position, red with slight purple tinge, small amount of dried blood, no rashes, no erythema, no ulcers, no fissures*
- Palpation: *firm lump, exquisitely tender, not warm, smooth regular borders, surrounding tissue and perineum soft and non-tender*
- Digital rectal examination: *unable to complete as too tender*

Investigations

BBMI-O: Bedside, **B**loods, **M**icrobiology, **I**maging and **O**ther

Investigation	Rationale
Bedside	
Bloods	
▧ FBC	▧ Looking for infection and anaemia
▧ CRP	▧ Looking for infection
Microbiology	
Imaging	
▧ CT pelvis	▧ Looking for evidence of malignancy within the anal canal, may also be useful to identify a fistula
▧ MRI pelvis	▧ Looking for evidence of perianal fistula and identifying the presence of a tract
Other	
▧ Proctoscopy / colonoscopy	▧ To directly visualise any abnormalities causing pain

Diagnosis

Haemorrhoids: external, pregnancy-induced

A firm, tender lump with smooth regular borders in correlation with the history is suggestive of haemorrhoids.

Anatomy

- ▧ The internal rectal venous plexus helps the anus mucous membrane to form three cushion-like masses in the 3, 7 and 11 o'clock positions, corresponding to the common sites for haemorrhoids, which are varicosities at these sites
- ▧ External haemorrhoids originate below the dentate line
- ▧ Internal haemorrhoids originate above the dentate line and are further classified into grades:
  - I – Bleeding, may protrude into but not prolapse out of the anal canal
  - II – Prolapse on defecation but reduce spontaneously
  - III – Require manual reduction
  - IV – Irreducible, permanently prolapsed

Haemorrhoids are often a diagnosis made on history and examination, investigations are only required for work-up of complications or to rule out more sinister causes of anal pain.

Management

Medical

▓ Aim to reduce swelling and manage pain:
- Ice pack to area
- Regular paracetamol and avoiding opioids
- Stool softeners
- Local anaesthetic gel
- Vasoactive cream / suppository

Prevention

▓ High-fibre diet
▓ Regular fluids to avoid dehydration
▓ Avoid straining and heavy lifting
▓ Usually haemorrhoids resolve post-partum

Interventions

▓ Better done when acute swelling improves
▓ Options:
- Lord's procedure:
  ▸ Anus dilatation to relieve anal spasm
- Sclerosing agent injecting:
  ▸ Triggers fibrosis and atrophy
  ▸ Can be done in outpatient clinic
  ▸ Usually requires multiple procedures every 4–6 weeks
- Rubber band ligation:
  ▸ Painful for at least 4–5 days
  ▸ May cause ulceration or delayed haemorrhage
  ▸ Can be done under local anaesthetic

- Haemorrhoidectomy:
  ▸ Excision and ligation of vascular roots
  ▸ Side effects: bleeding, infection, pain
- Infrared photocoagulation:
  ▸ Repeat therapy required
  ▸ Less painful, more expensive
- Cryotherapy:
  ▸ Liquid nitrogen application
  ▸ Less painful, perianal discharge common
- Doppler-guided haemorrhoidal artery ligation:
  ▸ Day procedure
  ▸ Artery directly ligated, reduced bleeding risk
- Surgery:
  ▸ Open (Milligan Morgan), Closed (Ferguson's technique), Whitehead's circumferential, Park's submucosal
  ▸ Clamp and cautery, staple, ligature or diathermy

Complications of haemorrhoids

▓ Thrombosis: appear purple, oedematous, extreme pain
▓ Strangulation
▓ Prolapse
▓ Anaemia

Other differential diagnoses

▓ Abscess
▓ Perianal fistula
▓ Anal cancer

Station 6 **Ankle swelling**

A 20-year-old man presents to the emergency department with right ankle pain and swelling.

Tasks

1 Take a history
2 Perform a physical examination

3 Describe appropriate investigations
4 List some differential diagnoses and their brief management

---

Differential diagnoses (VIITAMINC)

Vascular:
- Deep vein thrombosis (DVT)
- Cardiac failure

Infective:
- Septic arthritis
- Cellulitis
- Joint infection other than septic arthritis (e.g. Lyme disease, fungal, viral)
- Reactive arthritis
- Osteomyelitis

Inflammatory:
- Gout/pseudogout
- Osteoarthritis
- Bursitis
- Tenosynovitis
- Monoarticular inflammatory joint disease:
  - Juvenile idiopathic arthritis
  - Spondyloarthropathy
  - Systemic lupus erythematosus (SLE)
  - Psoriatic arthritis
  - Synovial disease
  - Foreign body synovitis
  - Haemarthrosis
  - Intermittent hydrathrosis

Traumatic:
- Fracture
- Dislocation
- Sprain

Autoimmune:
- Pancreatitis
- Inflammatory bowel disease

Metabolic:
- Paget's disease
- Liver failure
- Renal failure

Iatrogenic

Neoplastic:
- Malignancy – bone cancer, metastatic disease
- Lymphoma

Congenital

Other:
- Loose bodies

Before starting

Establish rapport:
- Introduce yourself
- Obtain consent to take a history and examine the patient
- Exposure: explain to the patient that you will need to do a lower limb examination which requires full exposure

Confirm patient details:
- Name — *Sunil Kohli*
- Age — *20 years*
- Occupation — *Student, athlete*

History

History of presenting complaint (SOCRATES)

- **S**ite: *right ankle pain and swelling*
- **O**nset: *worsening over 4 days after being tackled in a football game*
- **C**haracter: *dull ache, sharp when mobilising*
- **R**adiation: *none*
- **A**ssociated symptoms: *bruising surrounding the ankle*
- **T**ime: *constant*
- **E**xacerbating / relieving: *exacerbated by walking, relieved by rest, elevation and simple analgesia*
- **S**everity: *limiting day-to-day activities*

Past medical history and family history

- *Nil significant past medical history*
- *Nil family history*

Drug history and allergies

- *No known drug allergies*
- *Recent course oral antibiotics for ear infection*

Social history

- Smoking history: *non-smoker*
- Alcohol and drugs history: *social binge drinker, occasional marijuana use*
- *Plays football*
- *Studying construction management at technical and further education institution*

Examination

General inspection (ABCD-V)

- **A**ppearance: *patient looks well*
- **B**ody habitus: *normal, BMI 22*
- **C**ognition: *conscious and oriented*
- **D**evices / **D**rugs: *nil*
- **V**itals: *BP 123/78mmHg, HR 73bpm and regular; other vitals within normal limits; afebrile*

Lower limb

- Exposure:
  - *Lying supine on a completely flattened bed, both whole legs exposed (patient in underwear)*
- Inspection:
  - *Obvious asymmetry, right ankle more swollen than left, bruising over lateral and medial aspect of the right ankle, slightly warmer than left*
- Palpation:
  - *Tenderness over the right foot medial malleolus and forefoot, no pitting oedema bilaterally, no calf pain bilaterally*
- Movement:
  - Right ankle: *reduced active range of movement (ROM) eversion / inversion, plantar flexion and dorsiflexion due to pain, reduced passive ROM inversion / eversion, dorsiflexion 45 degrees and plantar flexion 45 degrees, limited again by pain*
  - Left ankle: *normal ROM passive and active*
  - Knees: *normal ROM passive and active bilaterally*

Investigations

BBMI-O: Bedside, **B**loods, **M**icrobiology, **I**maging and **O**ther

Investigation	Rationale
Bedside	
Bloods	
FBC	Looking for infection and anaemia
U&Es, calcium, CMP	Looking for renal function and calcium level in the setting of malignancy
CRP / ESR	Looking for signs of inflammation
Rheumatoid factor, HLA-B27, ANA	Screening for autoimmune disease
Microbiology	
Imaging	
X-ray ankle	Looking for a fracture or effusion, usually positive in osteoarthritis, crystal deposition, osteonecrosis, erosive arthritis, bone or marrow tumours, and can identify osteomyelitis
US ankle	Looking for effusion or foreign body, can also examine tendon sheaths
CT ankle	Good for looking at bones, fine fractures that may be missed
MRI ankle	Good at looking at soft tissues due to high anatomic resolution; can also assess chondral and bone alterations; consider if >8 weeks of pain
Other (in individuals where a diagnosis has not yet been made)	
Mantoux test	Screening for tuberculosis
Joint aspiration (arthrocentesis)	Can be done under US guidance; to get a sample of joint fluid and look for gout, pseudogout and infective causes

Decision whether to X-ray a foot can be made based on the Ottawa Ankle and Foot Rules, where X-rays are required if one of the following criteria is met:

Ankle	Foot
Bone tenderness along the distal 6cm of the posterior edge of the tibia or tip of the medial malleolus	Bone tenderness at the base of the fifth metatarsal
Bone tenderness along the distal 6cm of the posterior edge of the fibula or tip of the lateral malleolus	Bone tenderness at the navicular bone
Inability to bear weight for four steps	Inability to bear weight for four steps

Diagnosis

Ankle fracture

Classification

- Weber versus Lauge–Hansen:
  - Weber system focuses on the integrity of the syndesmosis which holds the ankle mortise together, whereas Lauge–Hansen focuses on the mechanism of injury:
    - Weber A: infra-syndesmotic = Lauge–Hansen supination adduction
    - Weber B: trans-syndesmotic = Lauge–Hansen supination external rotation
    - Weber C: supra-syndesmotic = Lauge–Hansen pronation external rotation
- Weber A:
  - Occurs below the syndesmosis which is intact
  - Resulting from an adducting force on a supinated foot
  - Tension on the lateral collateral ligaments results in rupture of the ligaments or avulsion of the lateral malleolus then a fracture of the medial malleolus
- Weber B:
  - At the level of the syndesmosis
  - Resulting from external rotation of the supinated foot
  - Rupture of the anterior syndesmosis → oblique fracture of the fibula → rupture of the posterior syndesmosis → avulsion of the medial malleolus (or medial collateral bands)
- Weber C:
  - Above the level of the syndesmosis
  - External rotation of the pronated foot
  - Avulsion of the medial malleolus → rupture anterior syndesmosis → fibular fracture (above level of syndesmosis) → avulsion of the posterior malleolus

Management

Non-operative

- Cast or CAM boot
- Indications:
  - Isolated non-displaced medial or lateral malleolus fracture <3mm displacement and no talar shift
  - Bimalleolus fracture if elderly or unable to undergo surgical intervention
  - Posterior malleolar fracture with <25% joint involvement

Operative

- ORIF: open reduction internal fixation
- Indications:
  - Any talar displacement
  - Isolated lateral or medial malleolar fracture with >3mm displacement
  - Bimalleolar fracture
  - Posterior malleolar fracture with >25% joint involvement
  - Bosworth fracture-dislocation
  - Open (compound) fractures
- Complications:
  - Wound problems
  - Deep infections
  - Malunion
  - Post-traumatic arthritis
  - Chronic regional pain syndrome

Other differential diagnoses

Fifth metatarsal fracture

- Often missed
- Involves:
  - An avulsion fracture (caused by plantar aponeurosis pull on the bony tuberosity), usually due to ankle inversion injury

- Jones fracture: at the base of the 4th and 5th metatarsals, due to a large adductive force to the foot while plantarflexed
- A shaft fracture: distal to the 5th metatarsal joint, often caused by stress, i.e. chronic overload

Navicular fracture

- On 'overuse' fracture, i.e. track and field athletes
- Predisposed to stress injuries as it is quite avascular
- Usually gradual onset of pain, mostly with exercise
- Ecchymosis and swelling often absent

Ankle sprain

Two types:
- High ankle sprain: 1–10% of sprains, syndesmosis injury
- Low ankle sprains:
  - ATFL (anterior talofibular ligament) injury:
    - Most common
    - Mechanism: plantar flexion and inversion
  - CFL (calcaneofibular ligament) injury:
    - Second most common
    - Mechanism: dorsiflexion and inversion

Classifications of low ankle sprain:

	Ligamentous disruption	Ecchymosis and swelling	Pain with weight bearing
Grade I	None	None	None
Grade II	Stretch (no tear)	Moderate	Mild
Grade III	Complete tear	Severe	Severe

Treatment:

- Non-operative:
  - **RICE: R**est, **I**ce, **C**ompression, **E**levation
  - Weight-bearing immobilisation in a walking boot or cast
  - Brace during strengthening exercises to prevent inversion and eversion
- Operative:
  - Anatomical reconstruction versus tendon transfer with tenodesis:
    - For Grades I–III that continue to have pain and instability or with bony avulsion
  - Arthroscopy:
    - Recurrent sprains and chronic pain caused by impingement

Station 7 **Axillary lump**

A 60-year-old woman presents to the GP with an axillary lump.

Tasks

1 Take a history
2 Perform a physical examination
3 Describe appropriate investigations
4 Formulate a management plan

Differential diagnoses (VIITAMINC)

Vascular

Infective:
- Reactive lymphadenopathy (due to secondary infection or allergic reaction)
- Tuberculosis (TB)
- Infected sebaceous cyst
- Folliculitis / hidradenitis suppurativa

Inflammatory:
- Ruptured infundibular follicular cyst
- Nodular fibromatosis
- Inflammatory rheumatoid lymphadenitis

Trauma

Autoimmune

Metabolic

Iatrogenic

Neoplastic:
- Lymphoma
- Breast carcinoma
- Metastatic carcinoma
- Leukaemia

Congenital

Other:
- Ectopic breast
- Lipoma

Before starting

Establish rapport:
- Introduce yourself
- Obtain consent to take a history and examine the patient
- Exposure: explain to the patient that you will need to do an axillary examination and likely breast examination; consider need for a chaperone

Confirm the patient details:
- Name   *Amy Black*
- Age   *60 years*
- Occupation   *Receptionist*

History

Lump history (SSSCHOMP)
- **S**ize: *bean size*
- **S**hape: *regular*
- **S**kin change / discharge: *no*
- **C**onsistency: *firm*
- **H**eat: *no*
- **O**nset: *noticed it yesterday in the shower, does not appear to be getting bigger*
- **M**obility: *mobile*
- **P**ain: *moderately painful*

Take a focused history
- Experienced this before: *no*

- Recent new antiperspirant / deodorant: *no*
- Contralateral or other lumps: *no*
- Breast changes / lumps / nipple discharge: *some redness, itchiness and pain around the left nipple*
- Systemic symptoms (fevers / sweats / rigors): *no*
- Recent injury (shaving / arm / hand): *no*
- Breast cancer risk factors: *yes, hormone replacement therapy (HRT)*
- Family history: *no*

Past medical and family history

- *Nil significant past medical history*
- *Nil family history*

Drug history and allergies

- *HRT*
- *NKDA*

Social history

- Smoking history: *non-smoker*
- Alcohol and drugs history: *non-drinker, nil illicit drugs*
- *Lives at home with husband and daughter*

Examination

General inspection (ABCD-V)

- **A**ppearance: *patient looks well*
- **B**ody habitus: *normal, BMI 22*
- **C**ognition: *conscious and oriented*
- **D**evices / **D**rugs: *nil*
- **V**itals: *BP 120/75mmHg, HR 75bpm and regular; other vitals within normal limits; afebrile*

Lump examination

- Position: *left axilla, anterior (pectoral) group*
- Size: *1.5 × 1.8cm*

- Shape: *round*
- Consistency: *firm*
- Mobility: *yes, skin moveable above lump*
- Skin changes: *no*
- Discharge: *no*
- Pain: *yes, on direct palpation*
- Number of lumps: *two, another smaller lump just inferior*

Axillary nodes examination

- *Patient to rest one arm completely on candidate's arm (e.g. patient's right arm on candidate's left arm to examine the right armpit)*
- Five places to examine:
  - Around the pectoralis muscles front and back: *normal front, palpation of two enlarged nodes at the back*
  - Around the upper arm muscles front and back: *normal*
  - The apex (lift patient's arm up, insert hand, let patient's arm down, wiggle fingers up a little higher): *normal*
- Examine the supraclavicular lymph nodes by asking patient to shrug shoulders: *normal*
- Examine the cervical, infraclavicular and parasternal lymph nodes: *normal*

Breast examination

- An essential task in the setting of an axillary lump
- General: *erythematous skin changes noted around the left areola, extending inferiorly to under the breast crease; hot to touch; no obvious dimpling of the skin, other skin changes; no nipple discharge or retraction*
- Palpation: *normal, no lumps palpated bilaterally; tenderness over the erythematous region; no tenderness on areolar palpation*

Investigations

BBMI-O: Bedside, **B**loods, **M**icrobiology, **I**maging and **O**ther

Investigation	Rationale
Bedside	
Bloods	
▨ FBC	▨ Looking for infection and anaemia and leukaemia

Investigation	Rationale
▨ CRP	▨ Looking for infection
▨ U&Es and creatinine	▨ Looking for electrolyte imbalances and renal injury
Microbiology	
▨ Swab MCS	▨ If nipple discharge is present, looking for signs of infection
Imaging	
▨ US of breast and axilla	▨ Looking for the number, size and consistency of lumps present
▨ Mammogram – breast	▨ Looking for lumps and calcification in the breasts
▨ CT chest	▨ Looking for characteristics of the lump, lymphadenopathy or any other lesions
Other	
▨ FNA biopsy	▨ Looking for histological diagnosis of tissue, common in breast cancer staging
▨ Core biopsy	▨ Looking for histological diagnosis of tissue, for cancer staging
▨ Excisional biopsy	▨ Gold standard if lymphoma or metastatic cancer suspected, results in the least amount of distortion of cell architecture

Diagnosis

Reactive lymphadenopathy secondary to areolar cellulitis

This is a clinical diagnosis, given an acute lump that is firm but mobile with surrounding erythema and surrounding lymphadenopathy.

The gold standard investigation to confirm reactive lymphadenopathy is clinical diagnosis. FBC/CRP can help confirm the diagnosis of inflammation/infection.

Management

Medical

▨ Analgesia as required
▨ IV flucloxacillin: to treat the cellulitis

Surgical

▨ Incision and drainage if lymphadenitis is present

Other differential diagnoses

▨ Folliculitis
▨ Hidradenitis suppurativa
▨ Sebaceous cyst

Station 8 **Back pain**

A 55-year-old man presents to the GP with a history of back pain.

Tasks

1 Take a history
2 Perform a targeted examination

3 Describe appropriate investigations
4 Formulate a management plan

Differential diagnoses (VIITAMINC)

Vascular:
- Abdominal aortic aneurysm (AAA)

Infective:
- Epidural abscess
- Vertebral osteomyelitis
- Pyelonephritis
- Pancreatitis
- Herpes zoster

Inflammatory:
- Spondylolysis
- Vertebral discitis
- Inflammatory spondyloarthropathy
- Renal colic
- Osteoarthritis
- Scoliosis
- Spinal canal stenosis
- Radiculopathy

Trauma:
- Trauma
- Herniated disc
- Back sprain
- Compression fracture

Autoimmune

Metabolic

Iatrogenic

Neoplastic:
- Bony metastases

Congenital

Other:
- Cauda equina syndrome

Before starting

Establish rapport:
- Introduce yourself
- Obtain consent to take a history and examine the patient
- Exposure: expose the patient adequately

Confirm the patient details:
- Name   *Sarfraz Rizwan*
- Age   *55 years*
- Occupation   *Architect*

History

History of presenting complaint (SOCRATES)

- **S**ite: *central lower back pain*
- **O**nset: *gradual*
- **C**haracter: *dull aching*
- **R**adiation: *down the right buttock and along the lateral side of the leg down to the foot*
- **A**ssociated symptoms: *7-day history of right foot numbness*
- **T**ime: *pain started 3 weeks ago, constantly there*

- **E**xacerbating / relieving: *worsened by bending and coughing*
- **S**everity: *limiting day-to-day activities*

Take a focused history

- Mode of onset: *bent over to pick up apartment plans*
- Symptoms in left leg: *nil*
- Weakness: *no*
- Difficulty walking: *yes*
- Paraesthesia / numbness: *right foot*
- Change in bowel habits: *nil change*
- Urinary retention: *no*
- Pain in other joints: *no*
- Fever / sweats / rigors: *no*
- History of malignancy: *no*
- Fatigue / loss of weight / night sweats: *no*
- History of trauma: *no*

Past medical history and family history

- *Nil significant past medical history*
- *No history of back pain / arthritis*
- *Nil family history*

Drug history and allergies

- *Nil regular medications*
- *NKDA*

Social history

- Smoking history: *1–2 cigarettes per day*
- Alcohol and drugs history: *one pint of beer per night, nil illicit drugs*
- *Works as a draughtsman*
- *Self-employed*

Examination

General inspection (ABCD-V)

- **A**ppearance: *patient looks in pain*
- **B**ody habitus: *overweight, BMI 28*
- **C**ognition: *conscious and oriented*
- **D**evices / **D**rugs: *nil*
- **V**itals: *BP 150/95mmHg, HR 95bpm; other vitals within normal limits*

Back

- Skin changes: *no*
- Asymmetry: *no*
- Lesions: *no*
- Palpable spinal pain: *no*
- *No skin changes in lower limbs*

Neurological examination

- *Difficulty standing on toes and heels to walk, walking otherwise well*
- Range of movement: *right ankle plantar flexion limited by pain, normal at all other joints bilaterally*
- Power / tone: *normal power and tone bilaterally*
- Sensation: *reduced over the right foot in the S1 distribution*
- Reflexes: *right ankle reflex reduced*
- Normal per rectum exam: *normal anal tone*
- *No saddle anaesthesia*
- *Straight leg raise test positive: elicited numbness in the right leg*

Investigations

BBMI-O: Bedside, **B**loods, **M**icrobiology, **I**maging and **O**ther

Investigation	Rationale
Bedside	
Urinalysis via dipstick	Looking for blood and the ability to urinate
Bloods	
FBC	Looking for infection and anaemia
CRP	Looking for infection

Investigation	Rationale
U&Es and creatinine	Looking for electrolyte imbalances and renal injury
LFTs / lipase	Looking for a source of back pain: hepatitis or pancreatitis?
Vitamin D	Looking for deficiency
Calcium level	Investigating for deficiency or malignancy
Microbiology	
Imaging	
Lumbosacral spine X-ray	Looking for arthritis or fractures in the spine
CT lumbosacral spine	Looking for infective or malignant processes
MRI spine	For examination of the intervertebral discs and spinal cords / nerve roots
Other	

Diagnosis

Prolapsed disc

A relatively benign history and positive straight leg raise test on examination leads to a likely diagnosis of a herniated disc.

The gold standard investigation to confirm prolapsed disc is an MRI spine.

Discussion

Most commonly occurs at L5 or S1. Symptoms may vary depending on the nerve root involved.

Presentation
- Back pain
- Radicular pain
- Cauda equina syndrome

Radiculopath
- A 'pinched nerve'
- Refers to a group of conditions whereby a nerve is dysfunctional (i.e. a neuropathy) where the problem occurs at the root of the nerve, shortly after it exits from the spinal cord
- This can include pain (radicular pain), weakness and numbness

- Sciatica is a type of radiculopathy – used to describe a sharp or burning pain radiating from the buttock down the back of the leg (along the path of the sciatic nerve)

Physical exam finding
- Ankle dorsiflexion (L4 or L5) and plantar flexion (S1) impaired – walk on heels / walk on toes
- Extensor hallicus longus weakness (L5) – difficulty elevating big toe against resistance
- Hip abduction weakness (L5 – gluteus medius) ± Trendelenburg gait
- Positive straight leg raise test – reproduces pain and paraesthesia by tensioning L5 and S1 nerves

Management

Non-operative

- Anti-inflammatories
- Rest and physiotherapy
- Nerve root corticosteroid injections – epidural or selective nerve block

Operative

- Microdiscectomy:
  - For persisting disabling pain that has failed conservative therapy ± weakness
  - Complications: dural tear, discitis and herniated nucleus pulposus

Other differential diagnoses

- Spinal cord or cauda equina compression
- Malignancy
- Spinal epidural abscess
- Vertebral compression fracture
- Lumbar spinal stenosis
- Ankylosing spondylitis

Station 9 **Breast lump**

A 55-year-old woman presents to the GP with a new breast lump.

Tasks

1 Take a history
2 Perform a physical examination
3 Describe appropriate investigations
4 Formulate a management plan

Differential diagnoses (VIITAMINC)

Vascular

Infective:
- Abscess
- Mastitis
- Tuberculosis (TB)

Inflammatory

Trauma:
- Haematoma

Autoimmune

Metabolic

Iatrogenic

Neoplastic:
- Benign:
  - Fibroadenoma

- Galactocele
- Phyllodes tumour
- Lipoma
- Breast cyst
- Intraductal papilloma
- Fibrocystic breasts
- Atypical ductal hyperplasia (ADH)
- Malignant:
  - Invasive lobular carcinoma
  - Invasive ductal carcinoma
  - Paget's disease
  - Inflammatory breast cancer
  - Ductal carcinoma *in situ* (DCIS)
  - Angiosarcoma

Congenital

Before starting

Establish rapport:
- Introduce yourself
- Obtain consent to take a history and examine the patient
- Exposure: explain to the patient that you will need to examine her breast and consider the need for a chaperone

Confirm patient details:
- Name — *Mary Sunderland*
- Age — *55 years*
- Occupation — *Personal assistant*

History

Lump history (SSSCHOMP)
- **S**ize: *2 × 2cm*
- **S**hape: *feels irregular*
- **S**kin changes / discharge: *no*
- **C**onsistency: *firm*
- **H**eat: *no*
- **O**nset: *first noticed 1 month ago when in bed*
- **M**obility: *no*
- **P**ain: *yes, a dull ache; can become sharp if you push on the area*

Breast cancer risk factors (very important to ascertain in breast lump cases)

- Family history:
  - Male: *no*
  - First-degree relative <40 years: *yes, mother aged 39 years*
  - Two first-degree relatives: *no*
- Increasing age:
  - >70 years = 26%
  - 50–69 years = 50% **high-risk group**
  - <50 years = 24%
- Previous breast cancer: *no*
- *BRCA1* and *BRCA2* genes present (66% chance of getting cancer): *not known*
- Obesity (due to increased oestrogen production): *yes, BMI 30*
- Hormone replacement therapy (HRT; over 5 years): *yes, HRT coming up 5 years this year*
- Caucasian: *yes*
- Previous history / family history of ovarian cancer: *no*

Protective factors (general decrease in oestrogen exposure)

- Early menopause: *no, menopause at 50 years*
- Pregnancy especially early: *no, first child at 30 years*
- Breastfeeding (6 months): *yes*
- Potentially alcohol and exercise: *yes, social drinker; no exercise*

Examination

General inspection (ABCD-V)

- **A**ppearance: *patient looks well*
- **B**ody habitus: *normal, BMI 21*
- **C**ognition: *conscious and oriented*
- **D**evices / **D**rugs: *nil*
- **V**itals: *BP 110/65mmHg, HR 63bpm and regular; other vitals within normal limits; afebrile*

Starting notes

- Avoid terms like 'look', 'feel', 'great', 'beautiful', 'expose'
- Use terms like 'check', 'examine', 'palpate'
- Consider the use of a chaperone in certain settings

Visual sitting

- Ask the patient to bring their gown down to their waist
- Ask the patient to follow your abduction of both arms at the same time and then back down
- As the arms come back down, ask the patient to put their hands on their hips and lean forward slightly
- Check the sides of the breasts while the patient does this
- Candidate should comment on presence of:
  - Skin dimpling: *no*
  - Asymmetry: *no*
  - Skin colour change: *no*
  - Nipple changes / inversion: *no*
  - Peau d'orange appearance (a sign of inflammatory breast cancer): *no*

Physical examination

- Ask the patient to lie down and lift their left / right arm up and rest it next to their head on the pillow
- Using the flats of your hands, starting on the posterior axillary line, fingers flat, movement from the shoulder, making sure straight lines are followed
- Moving hands in a circular motion: light circle, firm circle and then medium drag
- Warn the patient just before reaching the nipple area, as it might be sensitive
- Continue this all the way to the sternum and examine the sternum as well
- Do not forget to palpate over the sternum
- Lump:
  - Position: *right breast, 8 o'clock position, 4cm from the areola*
  - Size: *2 × 1.5cm*
  - Shape: *irregular*
  - Consistency: *firm*
  - Mobility: *immobile*
  - Skin changes: *no*
  - Discharge: *no*
  - Pain: *some discomfort on palpation, no acute pain*
  - Number of lumps: *one*

A breast examination must also include a lymph node examination

▨ Axillary nodes: *none palpable*
  ● Raise the patient's arm, using your left hand for their right side, palpating with the pulps of your fingers as high as possible into the axilla

  ● Palpate all five groups: central, lateral (above the scapula), pectoral (medial), infraclavicular and subscapular (most inferior)
▨ Supraclavicular nodes: *none palpable*
  ● Get the patient to shrug their shoulders, palpate above the clavicle

Investigations

BBMI-O: Bedside, **B**loods, **M**icrobiology, **I**maging and **O**ther

Investigation	Rationale
Bedside	
Bloods	
▨ FBC	▨ Looking for infection and anaemia
▨ CRP	▨ Looking for infection
Microbiology	
Imaging	
▨ Mammography	▨ Used as a screening and diagnostic tool in lump and calcification discovery; only applicable in over-35 age group
▨ US breast and axilla	▨ Looking for breast lumps
▨ MRI breast	▨ Utilised when multiple pockets of DCIS are found
▨ CT chest / abdomen / pelvis	▨ For staging in metastases; looking for the extent of spread
▨ PET scan	▨ For staging of cancer
Other	
▨ FNA cytology	▨ Looking for histological diagnosis of the breast lump
▨ Core biopsy	▨ Looking for the histological diagnosis of the breast lump

Diagnosis

Ductal carcinoma *in situ* (DCIS)

A firm, non-mobile lump in a 55-year-old woman is suspicious for malignancy; however, with a relatively benign examination it is likely to be in early stages.

The gold standard investigation to confirm breast cancer and histological type is a tissue sample, either by biopsy or excision.

Discussion

- Earliest form of breast cancer
- Itself is not invasive as the cancer cells have not spread outside the ducts; however, has the potential to become malignant
- May present as a lump or be asymptomatic and discovered during breast screening
- Seen best on mammograms as clusters of calcification
- May have hormone receptor tests conducted
- If many areas of DCIS suspected, MRI may be helpful in determining extent of disease

Tumour staging

Tumour size staging number	Diameter	Node involvement	Clinical stage
T1	T1a: 0–5mm	N0	I
	T1b: 5–10mm	N1	IIA
	T1c: 10–20mm	N2	IIIA
T2	20–50mm	N0	IIA
		N1	IIB
		N2	IIA
T3	>50mm	N0	IIB
		N1–2	IIIA
T4	Tumour involves skin or chest wall	N0–2	IIIB

Management

Medical
- Hormonal therapy: depends on the receptor status (oestrogen / progesterone positive or negative)
- Adjuvant radiotherapy: in conjunction with breast-conserving surgery (i.e. wide local excision) as a means to reduced tumour recurrence

Surgical
- Wide local excision
- Mastectomy – curative in over 98% of patients with DCIS:
  - Breast reconstruction: individual choice
  - Sentinel lymph node biopsy: although not routinely indicated in DCIS, if undertaking a mastectomy it is recommended as the ability to perform accurately post the procedure is impossible with the lymphatic drainage pattern alterations; patients who require mastectomies often have a higher likelihood of having an invasive cancer due to larger disease foci
- If DCIS covers a large area of the breast and is high grade, lymph node excision may be required:
  - Different levels of dissection depending on the bulk of disease
  - Identification and preservation of the long thoracic and thoracodorsal nerves essential
  - Dissection up to the axillary vein

Complication
Lymphoedema:
- A common complication of breast axillary surgery resulting in swelling of the ipsilateral

arm or increased oedema over the breast or torso
- Develops gradually, may result in numbness or tingling of the affected area
- Other symptoms including burning, aching and heaviness
- Important to avoid procedure of injury to the affected arm as infection risk is higher without the usual effective lymphatic drainage
- Treatment:
  - Sleeves, bandages and pumps to help lymph flow
  - Skin protection
  - Losing weight
  - Laser therapy

Breast lump differentials
- Fibroadenoma
- Breast cyst
- Phyllodes tumour
- Intraductal papilloma
- Invasive lobular / DCIS
- Paget's disease
- Inflammatory breast cancer
- Angiosarcoma

Station 10 **Chest pain**

A 25-year-old man presents to the emergency department with chest pain.

Tasks

1 Take a history
2 Perform a targeted examination

3 Describe appropriate investigations
4 Formulate a management plan

Differential diagnoses (VIITAMINC)

Vascular:
- Acute coronary syndrome
- Pulmonary embolism
- Thoracic aortic dissection
- Anaemia

Infective:
- Pneumonia
- Lung abscess
- Aspergilloma
- Tuberculosis (TB)
- Peptic ulcer disease

Inflammatory:
- Pericarditis
- Costochondritis
- Rib / sternal fracture
- Pneumonitis
- Exacerbation of asthma / chronic obstructive pulmonary disease (COPD)
- Pericardial effusion
- Gastritis

Trauma:
- Tension pneumothorax
- Pulmonary contusion
- Oesophageal perforation

Autoimmune

Metabolic

Iatrogenic

Neoplastic:
- Malignancy – lung
- Lymphoma

Congenital

Other:
- Arrhythmia
- Ingested foreign body
- Hiatus hernia
- Retrosternal goitre
- Thymoma
- Anxiety

Before starting

Establish rapport:
- Introduce yourself
- Obtain consent to take a history and examine the patient
- Exposure: explain to the patient that you will need to examine his chest with shirt off

Confirm patient details:
- Name   *Sam Jarvis*
- Age   *25 years*
- Occupation   *Music technician*

History

History of presenting complaint (SOCRATES)

- **S**ite: *right-sided anterior chest wall*
- **O**nset: *sudden, constant*
- **C**haracter: *sharp, worse with deep inspiration (pleuritic)*
- **R**adiation: *nil*
- **A**ssociated symptoms: *acute shortness of breath (SOB)*
- **T**ime: *started 2 hours ago*

- **E**xacerbating / relieving: *exacerbated by deep breathing*
- **S**everity: *limiting function due to breathing difficulty*

Take a focused history

- Cough: *no*
- Haemoptysis: *no*
- Wheeze: *no*
- Flu-like symptoms: *no*
- Fevers / night sweats: *no*
- Ankle swelling: *no*
- Palpitations: *no*
- Risk factors for gastritis / peptic ulcer disease: *smoker, likes spicy foods, no NSAIDs*
- Exertional chest pain in the past: *no*
- Risk factors for pulmonary embolism: *no recent travel, no recent hospital admissions / surgery, no exogenous oestrogen, no calf tenderness*
- Syncopal episodes: *no*
- Postnasal drip: *no*
- Neck swelling: *no*
- Hoarse or changed voice: *breathy voice currently*

Past medical history and family history

- *Childhood asthma, no hospital / ICU admissions*
- *Nil family history*

Drug history and allergies

- *Nil*
- *NKDA*

Social history

- Smoking history: *occasional cigarettes*
- Alcohol and drugs history: *social drinker, smokes marijuana daily*
- *Works as a music technician*

Examination

General inspection (ABCD-V)

- **A**ppearance: *patient has obvious laboured breathing*
- **B**ody habitus: *low–normal BMI, tall stature*
- **C**ognition: *conscious and oriented*
- **D**evices / **D**rugs: *nil*
- **V**itals: *BP 121/68mmHg, HR 85bpm, RR 24 breaths per minute; oxygen saturation at 95% on room air*

Positioning

- Patient lying at 45 degrees or sitting upright
- Ensure neck and chest are fully exposed to the waist

Respiratory

- Inspection:
  - Hands:
    - *No clubbing, peripheral cyanosis, nicotine staining, muscle wasting / weakness*
    - *No flapping tremor (asterixis)*
  - Face:
    - *Examination of the eyes, ears, nose, mouth are all unremarkable*
    - *No nasal polyps, engorged turbinates or enlarged tonsils*
  - Neck:
    - *Trachea: midline, hypermovement present, no tracheal tug visualised*
    - *No palpable goitre or cervical lymphadenopathy*
  - Chest inspection:
    - *Pectus excavatum present*
    - *Reduced movement right chest*
- Palpation:
  - *Reduced chest expansion right side*
  - *Apex beat palpable*
  - *Vocal fremitus hyporesonant right side*
- Percussion:
  - *Hyper-resonant to percussion upper aspect right chest*
- Auscultation:
  - *Reduced air entry right chest apex to midzone*
  - *No wheeze, no added sounds*
- Pemberton's sign: *negative*
  - Ask patient to lift their arms over their head and wait for 1 minute
  - Watching for development of facial plethora, cyanosis, inspiratory stridor and jugular venous pressure elevation
  - Plethora: too much blood in the circulatory system
  - Caused by superior vena cava obstruction due to a mass or goitre with retrosternal extension

Investigations

BBMI-O: **B**edside, **B**loods, **M**icrobiology, **I**maging and **O**ther

Investigation	Rationale
Bedside	
Bloods	
▨ FBC	▨ Looking for infection and anaemia
▨ CRP	▨ Looking for infection
▨ U&Es and creatinine	▨ Looking for electrolyte imbalances
Microbiology	
Imaging	
▨ CXR (PA and lateral views): inspiration / expiration study	▨ Looking to visualise the extent of lung collapse; worrying signs that indicate a tension pneumothorax include shift in trachea and mediastinum contralaterally
▨ CT chest	▨ More sensitive than CXR at detecting small pneumothoraces and bullae
Other	

Diagnosis

Right-sided pneumothorax

Reduced chest expansion, air entry and vocal fremitus with a hyper-resonant percussion note are highly suggestive of a pneumothorax.

The gold standard investigation to confirm a pneumothorax is an inspiration / expiration CXR, though if concerned that this may be a tension pneumothorax, investigations should not delay management.

Discussion

- ▨ The accumulation of air between the visceral and parietal pleura
- ▨ All pneumothoraces have the potential to become a tension pneumothorax
- ▨ Causes:
  - ● Idiopathic
  - ● Bullae:
    - ▸ Cyst-like outpouchings from the lung parenchyma with weak walls
    - ▸ Can be congenital or due to COPD / emphysema
  - ● Asthma
  - ● Traumatic:
    - ▸ Penetrating injury
    - ▸ Rib fracture
    - ▸ Chest trauma

Management

- ▨ Call for help
- ▨ Supplementary oxygen (nasal prongs if tolerated, otherwise upgrade to Hudson mask)
- ▨ IV access large bore (×2)

- Portable CXR (unless concerned for tension pneumothorax)
- Resuscitation / HDU cubicle
- Pulse oximetry
- Insertion of intercostal catheter

Indications for intercostal catheter (ICC)

- Pneumothorax
- Pleural effusion: diagnostic or therapeutic
- Haemothorax
- Postoperatively:
  - Lung resection / pneumonectomy
  - Oesophagectomy
  - Any operation in which the pleura may have been breached

Techniques

- US guided:
  - For a targeted insertion, particularly used for pockets of small fluid or collection
- Seldinger technique:
  - Using a guidewire with progressive dilatation of the incision up to the catheter size
- Open:
  - For emergency situations, open incision with finger dissection to the pleural cavity and insertion of tube

Tension pneumothorax

- Emergency chest decompression by insertion of a large bore cannula into the second intercostal space, mid-clavicular line

Pneumothorax

- Some can be managed conservatively with serial CXRs if they are small and asymptomatic

- Insertion of ICC in fifth intercostal space, mid-axillary line

Complications

- Bleeding:
  - The neurovascular bundle injury can occur as it runs under each rib
- Visceral injury:
  - Pulmonary haematoma
  - Pulmonary vein / artery injury
  - Insertion into the cardiac ventricle
- Infection:
  - Introduction of a foreign body into a sterile space always carries this risk, therefore it is done as a strictly sterile procedure
  - Wound infection
  - Empyema
- Bronchopleural fistula:
  - If put in too far
  - Difficult to manage
- Lung collapse:
  - If drain becomes blocked
- Reactive pulmonary oedema:
  - Causing worsening SOB, requiring diuresis
  - Occurs when the lung re-expands too rapidly if it has been compressed for a long period

Other differential diagnoses

- Pulmonary embolism

Station 11 **Clubbing**

A 72-year-old man has presented to his GP clinic as his partner has been commenting that his fingers have been growing in size.

Tasks

1 Take a history
2 Perform a targeted examination
3 Describe appropriate investigations
4 Formulate a management plan

Differential diagnoses (VIITAMINC)

Vascular:
- Congestive cardiac failure

Infective:
- Bronchiectasis
- Infective endocarditis

Inflammatory:
- Pulmonary fibrosis
- Asbestosis
- Chronic obstructive pulmonary disease (COPD)
- Sarcoidosis
- Inflammatory bowel disease

Trauma

Autoimmune

Metabolic:
- Liver cirrhosis

Iatrogenic

Neoplastic:
- Lung cancer

Congenital:
- Cystic fibrosis
- Tetralogy of Fallot
- Coeliac disease

Before starting

Establish rapport:
- Introduce yourself
- Obtain consent to take a history and examine the patient
- Exposure: when physical examination is required, he will be required to take off shirt / vest

Confirm patient details:
- Name   *Dwight York*
- Age   *72 years*
- Occupation   *Retired, previously worked in a train yard*

History

History of presenting complaint

- Onset: *noticed a few months ago, hasn't gone away; initially thought it was an infection, but antibiotics aren't working*
- Further description of nails: *"my nails have become huge; the ends of my fingers have become wider!"*
- Associated symptoms: *feeling short of breath lately, and started having some significant coughing as well over the past month*
- Constitutional symptoms: *no fevers, no rashes; has been losing some weight lately, but has been eating normally*

Take a focused history

- Shortness of breath: *yes, over the past few months*
- Chest pain: *no*
- Describe breathing: *more difficult recently; coughing a lot more lately*
- Cough: *yes, regularly over the past month; occasionally a little fleck of blood; "it's quite frightening now…"*
- Exacerbating / relieving factors: *no*
- Coughing / breathing worse on walking: *no*
- Pain relieved on sitting up: *no*
- Swelling in legs: *no swelling in legs*
- Syncopal episodes (fainting): *no*

Past medical history and family history

- *Nil known past medical history*
- *Father was a long-term smoker; he was never diagnosed with anything but occasionally coughed up blood like this too*

Drug history and allergies

- *Nil regular medications; has been taking a Ventolin puffer over the past couple of weeks*
- *NKDA*

Social history

- Smoking history: *40 pack-years*
- Alcohol and drugs history: *non-drinker, nil illicit drugs*
- *Lives at home with partner*

Examination

General inspection (ABCD-V)

- **A**ppearance: *patient looks comfortable; occasional dry cough*
- **B**ody habitus: *high BMI, 29*
- **C**ognition: *patient is conscious and oriented*
- **D**evices / **D**rugs: *has a Ventolin inhaler with no spacer; pack of cigarettes in pocket*
- **V**itals: *BP 130/90mmHg, HR 90bpm and regular, RR 20 per minute; oxygen saturation at 94% on room air; afebrile*

Chest

- Inspection: *no surgical scars or visible pulsations; barrel-chested individual; apex beat not visualised*
- Palpation: *apex beat not displaced, mid-clavicular 5th intercostal; no thrills or heaves felt*
- Percussion: *no effusions notable; no dullness to percussion at posterior chest*
- Auscultation: *dual heart sounds with no murmurs; quiet breath sounds globally; fine bi-basal crackles*

Abdomen

- Inspection:
- Palpation: *no tenderness in any area of the abdomen; no evidence of abdominal aortic aneurysm*
- Percussion: *no ascites or organomegaly*
- Auscultation: *no bruits; bowel sounds present*

Hand examination

- Inspection: *beaked nails; angle between nail bed and finger is lost – seems continuous; no erythema; no Osler's nodes / Janeway lesions*
- Palpation: *spongy nailbed area, otherwise normal examination; no tenderness*
- Movement: *full range of movement noted*

Investigations

BBMI-O: Bedside, **B**loods, **M**icrobiology, **I**maging and **O**ther

Investigation	Rationale
Bedside	
Bloods	
▨ FBC	▨ Looking for infection and anaemia
▨ CRP	▨ Looking for infection
▨ U&Es and creatinine	▨ Looking for electrolyte imbalances and renal injury
▨ Cardiac biomarkers	▨ Looking for myocardial infarction
▨ Venous blood gas	▨ Looking for baseline lung function, or propensity to retain carbon dioxide
▨ D-dimer	▨ Looking for increased risk of a clotting disorder
▨ Tumour markers for lung cancer (CEA, NSE, CYFRA 21-1)	▨ Looking for increased serum tumour markers suggestive of lung cancer
Microbiology	
Imaging	
▨ CXR (PA and lateral views)	▨ Looking for pulmonary infection and collapse; masses, pleural effusion and air bronchograms
▨ CT chest / abdomen / pelvis	▨ Looking for evidence of malignancy within thoracic cavity, lung, or abdomen; also can find anatomical abnormalities of lungs suggestive of interstitial pathology
Other	
▨ Transthoracic echocardiogram	▨ Looking for signs of cardiac dysfunction, potentially signalling a congenital abnormality
▨ Pulmonary function tests	▨ Looking for obstructive or restrictive defects associated with lung disease (could point to COPD / interstitial lung disease)

Diagnosis

Lung cancer

An insidious onset of clubbing, unintentional loss of weight and occasional haemoptysis in a patient with a heavy smoking history should raise suspicions for malignancy.

The gold standard investigation for lung cancer would be a CT chest with associated bronchoscopy + biopsy if a nodule is found.

Management

The treatment of lung cancer is highly dependent upon what type of cancer it is (via tissue biopsy) and what stage it is. A general summary will be described here.

Non-small cell lung cancer

As non-small cell lung cancer (NSCLC) has a propensity to present as large nodules or tumours within the lung, surgical options are explored early – transitioning to chemotherapy/radiotherapy regimes should it advance.

- Stage 0 (*in situ*)–II NSCLC:
  - Surgical management is recommended in these cases
  - Surgery can take the form of a segmentectomy, lobectomy or pneumonectomy (removal of the whole lung)
  - From stage IB onward usually a combination of both surgical management AND chemotherapy/radiotherapy would be used to increase curative rates
- Stage III NSCLC:
  - Surgical management is usually recommended; however, it has a lower chance of being curative at this point
  - Stage III suggests that the tumour has now spread to ipsilateral lymph nodes along the chest wall; in some cases these can be removed along with thoracic surgery to remove the tumour
  - Chemotherapy and radiotherapy now play a strong role in the treatment of this stage of lung cancer
- Stage IV NSCLC:
  - The most advanced form of the disease, stage IV NSCLC means that the cancer has now spread to other organs and areas of the body; it is no longer possible to surgically remove the tumour given the metastatic nature of the disease
  - Chemotherapy/radiotherapy for treatment, but also for palliative purposes, is usually instituted in this case to maintain the quality of life for the affected patient
  - Surgical:
    - Surgical management is rarely performed and would be considered outside the scope of usually suggested management at this level of training
    - Pulmonary embolectomy is currently a rare procedure with high mortality rates; it is only performed in the context of a massive or sub-massive pulmonary embolus

Small cell lung cancer

Small cell lung cancer (SCLC) follows a similar treatment pathway to NSCLC; however, it is more heavily dependent on chemotherapy/radiotherapy due to its anatomical typing.

As such, in general:

- Stage 0–I SCLC: treated primarily with surgical removal of the affected lobe of the lung with lobectomy
- Stage II–III: will require adjuvant chemotherapy/radiotherapy prior to surgery; however, in some cases surgery may not be appropriate
- Stage IV: palliative chemotherapy/radiotherapy is usually undertaken to relieve symptoms for the patient affected

Other differential diagnoses

- COPD

Station 12 **Constipation**

A 78-year-old man presents to the GP with a 2-week history of worsening constipation, not improving despite the prescription of laxatives.

Tasks

1 Take a history
2 Perform a targeted examination
3 Describe appropriate investigations
4 Formulate a management plan

Differential diagnoses (VIITAMINC)

Vascular

Infective

Inflammatory:
- Pseudo-obstruction
- Inflammatory bowel disease

Trauma

Autoimmune

Metabolic:
- Hypercalcaemia
- Hypothyroidism

Iatrogenic:
- Medication-induced constipation

Neoplastic:
- Bowel cancer

Congenital:
- Inguinal / femoral hernia
- Coeliac disease

Other:
- Large bowel obstruction
- Diet

Before starting

Establish rapport:
- Introduce yourself
- Obtain consent to take a history and examine the patient
- Expose the patient: when physical examination is required, it will require shirt / vest to be taken off

Confirm patient details:
- Name — *Gordon Crane*
- Age — *78 years*
- Occupation — *Retired, previously a construction worker*

History

History of presenting complaint
- Onset: *over the past 2 weeks*

- Pain: *no abdominal or rectal pain*
- Describe the look of your stool: *"hardened, like a brick honestly"*
- Blood in stool: *had an episode last week, but nothing since*
- Mucus in stool: *no*
- Change in bowel habit: *constipated for past 2 weeks; before this had a few days of diarrhoea*
- Recent change in diet: *no*
- Nausea / vomiting: *no*
- Early feelings of fullness (satiety): *no*
- Unexplained weight loss: *yes, lost about 10kg over past 3 months*
- Constitutional symptoms: *no fevers / rigors / chills*

Take a focused history
- Lethargy: *no*
- Decreased water intake: *no*
- Increased thirst: *no*

░ Increased frequency of urination: *no*

░ Bone pain: *no*

Past medical history and family history

░ *Nil significant past medical history*

░ *Father had a 'gut cancer'; mother had a lot of polyps in the rectum that needed surgery*

Drug history and allergies

░ *Not on opiates*

░ *NKDA*

Social history

░ Smoking history: *30 pack-years*

░ Alcohol and drugs history: *non-drinker, nil illicit drugs*

Examination

General inspection (ABCD-V)

░ **A**ppearance: *patient looks comfortable*

░ **B**ody habitus: *overweight, BMI 28*

░ **C**ognition: *patient is conscious and oriented*

░ **D**evices / **D**rugs: *nil*

░ **V**itals: *BP 130/70mmHg; HR 70bpm and regular; afebrile*

Abdomen

░ Inspection: *no surgical scars, deformities or visible pulsations; no spider naevi, no significant bruising noted*

░ Palpation: *soft abdomen in all four quadrants; no tenderness; mass mildly palpable in left lower quadrant, difficult to characterise; no expansile abdominal aorta; no hernias notable while patient standing at femoral / inguinal areas*

░ Percussion: *no shifting dullness; no organomegaly*

░ Auscultation: *normal bowel sounds in all four quadrants; no renal bruits*

Digital rectal examination (DRE)

░ The candidate should obtain EXPLICIT consent before performing a DRE; if the patient is of the opposite sex, endeavour to have a chaperone at all times; a chaperone should always be offered to the patient prior to the examination

░ Inspection: *no external anal masses; no anal fissures / tears; no haemorrhoids*

░ Palpation: *no masses noted; no blood on finger – empty rectum; prostate normal calibre and size*

Investigations

BBMI-O: Bedside, **B**loods, **M**icrobiology, **I**maging and **O**ther

Investigation	Rationale
Bedside	
Bloods	
░ FBC	░ Looking for infection and anaemia
░ CRP	░ Looking for infection / inflammation
░ U&Es and creatinine	░ Looking for electrolyte imbalances and renal injury
░ Tumour markers (CEA / CA19-9)	░ Looking for raised serum levels to suggest the development of colorectal cancer
Microbiology	
Imaging	
░ AXR (PA and lateral views)	░ Looking for evidence of faecal loading, or dilated bowel loops
░ CT abdomen / pelvis	░ Looking for evidence of colonic masses, intra-abdominal collections, metastases, hernias

Investigation	Rationale
Other	
▨ Colonoscopy ± biopsies	▨ Looking for areas of thickened bowel wall, inflamed bowel wall; positive biopsies would be indicative of malignancy

Diagnosis

Bowel cancer

A relatively benign abdominal examination with insidious onset of symptoms associated with unintentional weight loss is highly suspicious for malignancy.

The gold standard investigation to confirm bowel cancer is colonoscopy with a positive biopsy.

Management

Treatment for bowel cancer is highly dependent on the stage of the cancer. Cases are usually discussed through a multidisciplinary meeting to determine the correct course of treatment.

Medical

▨ Supportive measures such as analgesia, laxatives, and anti-emetics should be prescribed to reduce pain and allow the passage of softer stool
▨ The patient should be referred to a colorectal specialist for further guidance on management
▨ Chemotherapy/radiotherapy can be considered with appropriately staged colorectal cancer, in both the neoadjuvant and adjuvant setting

Surgical

▨ Surgical management is common for colorectal cancer and depending on the location of the tumour would normally involve an excision of the tumour, with a wide area of normal bowel taken as well
▨ This could take the form of a hemicolectomy, (ultra) low anterior resection or total colectomy

Colorectal cancer is a significant diagnosis with a long treatment pathway. The symptoms that may present in early-stage colorectal cancer involve blood in stool, changes in bowel habit (fluctuating between diarrhoea/constipation) and constitutional symptoms such as unexplained weight loss. Eventually development of colorectal cancer, if left untreated, can result in partial or complete large bowel obstruction. Metastatic disease follows this, leading to seeding within the abdomen and functions of the liver, kidneys and stomach can be affected depending on where the metastatic deposits lie.

Staging

Staging of colorectal cancer is dependent on imaging results, and biopsy via colonoscopy.

▨ Stage 0 (carcinoma *in situ*) – would usually present as a polyp, hence polypectomy and/or local excision of the tumour can be undertaken; this can be done via colonoscopy
▨ Stage 1 – bowel resection with primary anastomosis is considered at this stage; chemotherapy/radiotherapy is usually not indicated
▨ Stages 2 and 3 – usually involves a combination of bowel resection ± the formation of a stoma, alongside adjunct chemotherapy/radiotherapy soon after; if there are clear margins and the cancer is seen to be in remission, then reversal of the formed stoma can be completed months after the initial surgery
▨ Stage 4 – this stage implies that there are metastatic deposits; surgery, in this case,

is usually of a palliative nature to relieve obstruction or excessive abdominal pain.

Chemotherapy and radiotherapy are commonly first line in these circumstances to help reduce the size of the affecting tumours and to help relieve symptoms. Palliative care management can be considered in late-stage colorectal cancer where none of the above treatment options would be considered to have considerable benefit.

Other differential diagnoses

- Inguinal / femoral hernia
- Large bowel obstruction

Station 13 **Cough**

An 18-year-old woman presents to the ENT clinic with a 3-day history of a cough.

Tasks

1 Take a history
2 Perform a physical examination

3 Describe appropriate investigations
4 Formulate a management plan

Differential diagnoses (VIITAMINC)

Vascular

Infective:
- Tonsillitis
- Pharyngitis
- Peritonsillar abscess (quinsy)
- Epstein–Barr virus (EBV; glandular fever)
- Bronchitis
- Pneumonia
- Pertussis
- Bronchiectasis

Inflammatory:
- Asthma

- Gastro-oesophageal reflux disease (GORD)
- Gastritis

Trauma

Autoimmune

Metabolic

Iatrogenic

Neoplastic

Congenital

Other:
- Foreign body

Before starting

Establish rapport:
- Introduce yourself
- Obtain consent to take a history and examine the patient
- Exposure: when physical examination is required, it will require top/vest to be taken off

Confirm patient details:
- Name — *Catriona McDowell*
- Age — *18 years*
- Occupation — *High school student*

History

History of presenting complaint
- Onset: *worsening over the last 3 days*

- Pain: *"yes, in the back of my throat; has also been worsening over the past couple of days; dull in character, worse when I cough"*
- Radiation: *no*
- Exacerbating/relieving factors: *"taking paracetamol and ibuprofen helps; last time this happened I took antibiotics and things got better"*
- Associated symptoms: *"feels like there is a lump in the back of my throat"*
- Change in taste/hearing: *no*
- Difficulty opening/closing mouth: *no*
- Sputum: *no*
- Blood: *no*
- Rashes: *no*
- Has this ever happened before: *"yes, this is the third time in the past month; I had something like this quite regularly as a kid too"*
- Constitutional symptoms: *no fevers/weight loss*

hold

Past medical history and family history

- Nil significant past medical history
- Family history: nil

Drug history and allergies

- No regular medications; paracetamol and ibuprofen PRN
- NKDA

Social history

- Smoking history: non-smoker
- Alcohol and drugs history: non-drinker, nil illicit drugs

Examination

General inspection (ABCD-V)

- **A**ppearance: patient looks comfortable
- **B**ody habitus: normal, BMI 20
- **C**ognition: patient is conscious and oriented
- **D**evices / **D**rugs: nil
- **V**itals: BP 120/80mmHg, HR 60bpm and regular; afebrile

ENT examination

- Inspection:
  - Ear: no evident masses, no erythema, no discharge
  - Nose: normal inspection, no septal deviation, no discharge from nose
  - Throat: reddened back of throat; small plaque associated with right tonsillar inflammation; no evident abscess formation; gag reflex present
- Palpation:
  - Ear: no mastoid tenderness; skin not hot to touch
  - Nose: no evident deformity; no fractures

Chest

- Inspection: no surgical scars, deformities or visible pulsations; apex beat not visualised
- Palpation: apex beat not displaced, mid-clavicular 5th intercostal; no thrills or heaves are felt
- Percussion: no effusions notable; no dullness to percussion at posterior chest
- Auscultation: dual heart sounds with no murmurs; good air entry with symmetrical breath sounds; no added sounds

Investigations

BBMI-O: Bedside, **B**loods, **M**icrobiology, **I**maging and **O**ther

Investigation	Rationale
Bedside	
Bloods	
FBC	Looking for infection and anaemia
CRP	Looking for infection / inflammation
U&Es and creatinine	Looking for electrolyte imbalances and renal injury
Microbiology	
Throat swab for MCS	Looking for bacterial growth in tonsillar plaque
Nasopharyngeal aspirate	To check for viral pathogens

Investigation	Rationale
Imaging	
▨ CT facial sinuses	▨ Looking for opacification of facial sinuses and evidence of inflammation
Other	

Diagnosis

Tonsillitis

An inflamed tonsil with associated white patches in a well-looking patient with a history of similar episodes in the past should raise suspicion for tonsillitis.

Management

Treatment for tonsillitis is rarely surgical; however, recurrent cases or those in the paediatric population can benefit from surgical management. Tonsillitis is more commonly due to a viral pathogen, though can also be due to bacteria. Otherwise, treatment is as described below.

Medical

- ▨ Supportive measures such as analgesia, including paracetamol and ibuprofen, can assist in supportive management of tonsillitis
- ▨ Antibiotic therapy can be indicated in cases showing high fever, or those not responding to conservative management; the majority of bacterial pathogens causing tonsillitis are due to *Streptococcus* spp. and as such penicillins, including phenoxymethylpenicillin or amoxicillin, are indicated

Be wary of using amoxicillin, however, as EBV can mimic the above symptoms and a widespread rash can occur if this is treated with amoxicillin.

Surgical

- ▨ Tonsillectomy can be performed in cases of recurrent tonsillitis; it is usually performed in the paediatric population to prevent further attacks or the development of a peritonsillar abscess
- ▨ Current recommendations suggest tonsillectomy in the event of at least seven episodes within 1 year or at least five episodes per year for 2 years
- ▨ The above scenario shows an 18-year-old woman with tonsillitis – this is infrequent but does occur in the general populace; usually, after childhood the size of tonsils regress, and as such tonsillitis becomes less common; at this age surgical management would not be recommended without recurring history of severe tonsillitis

Other differential diagnoses

- ▨ Peritonsillar abscess (quinsy)
- ▨ EBV (glandular fever)

Station 14 **Cyanosis**

A 63-year-old man presents to his cardiologist for a regular check-up. He has been noticing some pain in his legs lately and the colour of his legs has been changing too.

Tasks

1 Take a history
2 Perform a physical examination

3 Describe appropriate investigations
4 Formulate a management plan

Differential diagnoses (VIITAMINC)

Vascular:
- Peripheral vascular disease
- Arterial thrombosis
- Large deep vein thrombosis (DVT)
- Left ventricular heart failure
- Severe aortic stenosis
- Anaemia
- Pulmonary embolism

Infective

Inflammatory:
- Raynaud's phenomenon

Trauma

Autoimmune

Metabolic

Iatrogenic

Neoplastic

Congenital

Other

Before starting

Establish rapport
- Introduce yourself
- Obtain consent to take a history and examine the patient
- Exposure: when physical examination is required, it will require shirt / vest and pants to be taken off

Confirm patient details:
- Name   *Jarrod Jennings*
- Age   *63 years*
- Occupation   *Shopkeeper; owns a coffee shop; currently working*

History

History of presenting complaint
- Onset: *last few weeks*

- Description of pain: *feels like a dull throbbing; worse further down legs, almost at feet*
- Change in colour: *legs become purple / blueish when walking; gets better when legs are put up or after resting*
- Both legs or one: *both legs*
- Associated symptoms: *has become slightly more tired than before; but nothing else; no shortness of breath*
- Swelling in legs: *no*
- Chest pain: *no*
- Orthopnoea: *no*
- Has this ever happened before: *no, this is new*
- Syncopal episodes: *no*
- Constitutional symptoms: *no fevers / rigors / chills*

Respiratory history
- Shortness of breath: *no*
- Cough: *no*

Past medical history and family history

- Medical history: *heart attack 2 years ago, type 2 diabetes, hypercholesterolaemia*
- Family history: *father died of heart attack at age 65 years*

Drug history and allergies

- *Aspirin 100mg daily and simvastatin 40mg daily*
- *NKDA*

Social history

- Smoking history: *20 pack-years*
- Alcohol and drugs history: *non-drinker, nil illicit drugs*

Examination

General inspection (ABCD-V)

- **A**ppearance: *patient looks comfortable*
- **B**ody habitus: *obese, BMI 32*
- **C**ognition: *patient is conscious and oriented*
- **D**evices/**D**rugs: *has a packet of cigarettes next to him*

- **V**itals: *BP 150/95mmHg; HR 90bpm and regular, RR 18 per minute; oxygen saturation at 96% on room air; afebrile*

Chest

- Inspection: *no surgical scars, deformities or visible pulsations; apex beat not visualised*
- Palpation: *apex beat displaced, mid-clavicular 6th intercostal; no thrills or heaves are felt*
- Percussion: *no effusions notable; no dullness to percussion at posterior chest*
- Auscultation: *dual heart sounds with no murmurs; good air entry with symmetrical breath sounds; no added sounds*

Lower limb examination

- Inspection: *both legs have no hair below the knee; no erythema, no swelling; at the level of feet, there is mild discoloration*
- Palpation: *cool feet to touch bilaterally; capillary refill between 2 and 3 seconds; dorsalis pedis and posterior tibial pulses are felt, though weak*
- Movement: *full range of movement noted*

Investigations

BBMI-O: Bedside, **B**loods, **M**icrobiology, **I**maging and **O**ther

Investigation	Rationale
Bedside	
Bloods	
FBC	Looking for infection and anaemia
CRP	Looking for infection
U&Es and creatinine	Looking for electrolyte imbalances
Cardiac biomarkers	Looking for myocardial infarction
Lipid profile	Looking for high cholesterol
D-dimer	Looking for increased risk of a clotting disorder

Investigation	Rationale
Microbiology	
Imaging	
▨ CXR (PA and lateral views)	▨ Looking for pulmonary infection and collapse; pleural effusion, and air bronchograms
▨ Duplex US lower limbs	▨ Looking for stenosis of lower limb arteries or lower limb vein thrombosis
▨ CT angiogram lower limbs	▨ Looking for signs of reduced perfusion to lower limbs and stenosis of lower limb arteries
▨ Ventilation / perfusion lung (VQ) scan	▨ Looking for signs of ventilation / perfusion mismatch, potentially leading to a diagnosis of pulmonary embolism (PE)
Other	
▨ ECG	▨ Looking for ECG changes associated with myocardial ischaemia, pericarditis or PE
▨ Echocardiogram	▨ Looking for signs of left-sided heart failure, or anatomical abnormalities of the heart

Diagnosis

Peripheral vascular disease

It is commonly a chronic disease, due to atherosclerotic changes of the limb arteries. The presence of diabetes and a smoking history worsens the pathology.

Acute cases of peripheral vascular disease are due to obstructive causes – either arterial thrombosis or large venous thrombosis.

The gold standard investigations to confirm lower limb peripheral vascular disease are a combination of duplex US and CT angiography of the lower limbs.

Management

Medical

▨ Supportive measures are limited; however, keeping the legs warm can be beneficial to allow for vasodilatation; cessation of smoking is important
▨ Control of diabetes and hypercholesterolaemia with medication is also necessary to prevent worsening

▨ In the event of thrombosis, anticoagulation can be used in the form of low molecular weight heparin, or a direct oral anticoagulant
▨ In the event of acute arterial thrombosis (would be a single limb pathology), then thrombolysis can be considered, but will usually proceed to surgical management

Surgical

Surgical management is centred around revascularisation of the affected legs:

- Angioplasty is performed to alleviate obstruction of affected vessels by the process of atherosclerosis; this is a minimally invasive, endovascular procedure; one leg is usually chosen for intervention at a time, as there is a risk of leg ischaemia should there be any complications; a stent can be placed inside the vessel during this procedure to ensure it remains patent
- Embolectomy can be performed in the case of acute peripheral vascular disease secondary to arterial thrombosis; in these cases, the affected leg is considered to have a compromised blood supply and the vasculature must be salvaged as soon as possible to prevent necrosis; the affected artery is identified via an intraoperative US or angiography, and the artery is opened and explored; the thrombus is then removed; the patient will then require a period of inpatient observation and will remain on therapeutic anticoagulation for 3–6 months postoperatively; in the event that extensive necrosis has already occurred due to a long period of time elapsing prior to surgery, then amputation of the affected limb may be required

Other differential diagnoses

- DVT
- Arterial thrombosis

Station 15 **Diarrhoea**

A 45-year-old woman presents to the general surgery outpatient clinic with a 1-week history of diarrhoea, not improving despite the prescription of loperamide (an antidiarrhoeal agent).

Tasks

1 Take a history
2 Perform a physical examination
3 Describe appropriate investigations
4 Formulate a management plan

Differential diagnoses (VIITAMINC)

Vascular:
- Ischaemic colitis

Infective:
- Diverticulitis
- Infective colitis
- Gastroenteritis

Inflammatory:
- Inflammatory bowel disease
- Irritable bowel syndrome
- Inflammatory colitis

Trauma

Autoimmune

Metabolic:
- Hyperthyroidism
- Electrolyte disturbance

Iatrogenic:
- Pseudomembranous colitis
- Medication-induced diarrhoea

Neoplastic

Congenital:
- Coeliac disease

Other:
- Diet-related

Before starting

Establish rapport:
- Introduce yourself
- Obtain consent to take a history and examine the patient
- Exposure: when physical examination is required, it will require top/vest to be taken off

Confirm patient details:
- Name — *Lucy Wilde*
- Age — *45 years*
- Occupation — *Lawyer, currently working*

History

History of presenting complaint

- Onset: *over the past week*
- Pain: *yes, abdominal pain in the left lower abdomen*
- Changes in bowel habit: *7–10 motions per day, increasing in the past couple of days*
- Blood in stool: *no blood seen*
- Mucus in stool: *"seems a bit mucous"*
- Recent change in diet: *no*
- Vomiting: *no*
- Early feelings of fullness (satiety): *no*
- Loss of appetite: *yes, past couple of days*
- Unexplained weight loss: *no*
- Constitutional symptoms: *fevers at home, on and off again; improved with paracetamol*

Take a focused history

- Lethargy: *no*
- Decreased water intake: *yes, due to pain*
- Increased thirst: *yes, but has not been drinking much*
- Increased frequency of urination: *no*
- Bone pain: *no*

Past medical history and family history

- *Nil significant past medical history*
- *Nil family history*

Drug history and allergies

- *No regular medications*
- *NKDA*

Social history

- Smoking history: *yes, but minimal; occasional cigarette*
- Alcohol and drugs history: *non-drinker, nil illicit drugs*

Examination

General inspection (ABCD-V)

- **A**ppearance: *patient looks comfortable*
- **B**ody habitus: *normal, BMI 22*
- **C**ognition: *patient is conscious and oriented*

- **D**evices / **D**rugs: *nil*
- **V**itals: *BP 110/70mmHg; HR 60bpm and regular; mild fever at 37.7°C*

Abdomen

- Inspection: *no surgical scars, deformities or visible pulsations; no spider naevi, no significant bruising noted*
- Palpation: *soft abdomen in all four quadrants; tenderness in left lower quadrant with mild rebound tenderness; no masses palpable; no expansile abdominal aorta; no hernias notable while patient standing at femoral / inguinal areas*
- Percussion: *no percussion tenderness; no shifting dullness; no organomegaly*
- Auscultation: *normal bowel sounds all four quadrants; no renal bruits*

Digital rectal examination (DRE)

The candidate should obtain EXPLICIT consent before performing a DRE; if the patient is of the opposite sex, endeavour to have a chaperone at all times; a chaperone should always be offered to the patient prior to examination

- Inspection: *no external anal masses; no anal fissures / tears; no haemorrhoids*
- Palpation: *no masses noted; no blood on finger; empty rectum*

Investigations

BBMI-O: Bedside, **B**loods, **M**icrobiology, **I**maging and **O**ther

Investigation	Rationale
Bedside	
Bloods	
FBC	Looking for infection and anaemia
CRP	Looking for infection / inflammation
U&Es and creatinine	Looking for electrolyte imbalances and renal injury
Tumour markers (CEA / CA19-9)	Looking for raised serum levels to suggest the development of colorectal cancer

Investigation	Rationale
Microbiology	
Blood cultures	Looking for bacteraemia
Faecal MCS	Looking for bacteria in stool
Faecal multiplex PCR + C. difficile toxin	Looking for evidence of C. difficile
Imaging	
AXR (PA and lateral views)	Looking for evidence of faecal loading, or dilated bowel loops
CT abdomen / pelvis	Looking for evidence of colonic masses, intra-abdominal abscess / inflammatory thickening of colon, hernias
Other	
In individuals where a diagnosis has not yet been made: • Colonoscopy ± biopsies (not usually performed in the acute phase for diverticulitis)	• Looking for areas of thickened bowel wall, inflamed bowel wall; a positive biopsy would be indicative of malignancy

Diagnosis

Diverticulitis

Left iliac fossa (LIF) pain and tenderness with clinical signs of an underlying infective process (fevers, mucus in stool) should raise suspicion for diverticulitis.

The gold standard investigation to confirm diverticulitis is a contrast CT abdomen / pelvis scan.

Discussion

Diverticulitis is a common diagnosis with a wide spectrum in regard to its effect on the human body. Its symptomatology can range from mild abdominal pain to sepsis, with a major complication of untreated diverticulitis being perforation.

A colonic diverticulum is a small outpouching of bowel found within the colon. It occurs generally due to weakening in the wall of colon, thought to be secondary to vigorous peristalsis of the colon. Age is a known risk factor, with incidence of diverticulitis up to approximately 50% in those above the age of 65 years.

Inflammation of diverticula leads to diverticulitis, with gut bacteria making up the most likely pathogens. As such antibiotic therapy is generally first line for any cases that are not classified as mild, or are not improving with simple diet restriction.

Colon wall can become friable due to inflammation, and as such can be at a greatly increased risk of perforation. If a diverticulum does perforate this can lead to the severe symptomatology that makes up 'The Acute Abdomen' and requires definitive surgical management to excise the perforated bowel, and repair the remaining healthy bowel.

Management

Treatment for diverticulitis is generally medical in nature, with surgical cases only if there is evidence of perforation, established collections (abscess), or in recurrent cases of diverticulitis.

Medical

- Diet restriction to clear fluids, this should continue until patient is able to tolerate clear fluids without pain, then slow upgrade
- Antibiotic regime; if pain not severe and able to tolerate in community, then oral antibiotics in the form of cefalexin / metronidazole should be considered; if ongoing fever / tachycardia or moderate abdominal pain, should be admitted to a hospital for intravenous antibiotics
- Analgesia
- Anti-emetics

Surgical

- Surgical management is reserved for perforated diverticulitis, chronic cases of diverticulitis, or where a diverticular abscess is proven
- In these cases the affected bowel, as well as a small amount of healthy bowel around will be taken; this may take the form of a hemicolectomy depending on the length of affected bowel
- Colonoscopy should be performed 6–8 weeks following an acute episode of diverticulitis to look for underlying lesions that may precipitate infective episodes

Other differential diagnoses

- Colitis (infective / inflammatory / ischaemic / pseudomembranous)

Station 16 **Dizziness**

A 28-year-old woman presents to the ENT clinic with a history of dizziness and lethargy, worsening over the past 3 months.

Tasks

1 Take a history
2 Perform a physical examination

3 Describe appropriate investigations
4 Formulate a management plan

Differential diagnoses (VIITAMINC)

Vascular:
- Orthostatic hypotension
- Anaemia

Infective

Inflammatory:
- Vestibular neuronitis
- Labyrinthitis
- Ménière's disease

Trauma

Autoimmune

Metabolic

Iatrogenic

Neoplastic:
- Vestibular schwannoma
- Intracranial lesion / tumour

Congenital

Other:
- Benign paroxysmal positional vertigo (BPPV)
- Arrhythmia
- Vasovagal syncope

Before starting

Establish rapport:
- Introduce yourself
- Obtain consent to take a history and examine the patient
- Exposure: expose the patient as appropriate

Confirm patient details:
- Name   *Harriet Summerskill*
- Age   *28 years*
- Occupation   *School teacher*

History

History of presenting complaint
- Onset: *very occasional, over past 3 months*
- Headache: *no*
- When does the dizziness occur: *"mostly when getting up from lying down"*

- Exacerbating / relieving factors: *"nothing really; I find it's worse if I don't drink enough water during the day"*
- Associated symptoms: *"I've been very tired over the past few months; nothing seems to make it better; I'm not sure if it is relevant, but my periods have been heavier than usual over the past months"*
- Any change in hearing: *no*
- Any discharge from ear: *no*
- Has this ever happened before: *no, not really*
- Constitutional symptoms: *no weight loss / fevers / rashes*

Gynaecological history
- Menstrual cycle: *regular, every 28 days, and lasts for 5 days*
- How many pads / tampons do you use: *"well for the first 2 days I have to change my pad every 1–2 hours; then it settles down afterwards"*

Have your periods always been heavy: *"no, has been like this for around 4–5 months; I don't know what's changed"*

Any clots: *no*

Vaginal discharge: *no*

Any chance you could be pregnant: *definitely not*

Are you currently menstruating: *no, due in 2 weeks*

Past medical history and family history

Nil significant past medical history

Nil family history

Drug history and allergies

No regular medications; not on oral contraceptive pill

NKDA

Social history

Smoking history: *non-smoker*

Alcohol and drugs history: *non-drinker, nil illicit drugs*

Diet: *"vegetarian, but I take mineral supplements as well"*

Examination

General inspection (ABCD-V)

Appearance: *patient looks comfortable*

Body habitus: *normal, BMI 20*

Cognition: *patient is conscious and oriented*

Devices / **D**rugs: *nil*

Vitals: *BP 110/70mmHg, HR 70bpm and regular; afebrile*

ENT examination

Inspection:
- Ear: *no discharge, no cellulitis, no erythema*
- Nose: *normal inspection, no septal deviation, no discharge from nose*
- Throat: *normal examination; no evident tonsillitis*

Palpation:
- Ear: *no mastoid tenderness; skin not hot to touch*
- Nose: *no evident deformity; no fractures*

Otoscopy:
- *No effusion at tympanic membranes bilaterally; normal examination*

Cranial nerve examination

All cranial nerves from I to XII are considered normal for this examination; no evident nerve palsy or abnormalities otherwise

Abdomen

Inspection: *no surgical scars, deformities, or visible pulsations; no spider naevi, no significant bruising noted*

Palpation: *soft abdomen in all four quadrants; no tenderness; no expansile abdominal aorta; no hernias notable at femoral / inguinal areas while patient standing*

Percussion: *no shifting dullness; no organomegaly*

Auscultation: *normal bowel sounds all four quadrants; no renal bruits*

Digital rectal examination and per vaginal examinations can be considered in this scenario with a chaperone escorting. In this case both examinations are normal

Investigations

BBMI-O: Bedside, **B**loods, **M**icrobiology, **I**maging and **O**ther

Investigation	Rationale
Bedside	
Bloods	
FBC	Looking for infection and anaemia
CRP	Looking for infection / inflammation
U&Es and creatinine	Looking for electrolyte imbalances and renal injury

Investigation	Rationale
▩ Iron levels	▩ Looking for iron deficiency, suggesting anaemia
▩ B$_{12}$ / folate levels	▩ Looking for B$_{12}$ / folate deficiency, suggesting anaemia
▩ Liver function tests	▩ Looking for increased bilirubin levels, suggestive of increased red blood cell breakdown
Microbiology	
Imaging	
Other	
▩ Uteroscopy	▩ Looking for uterine polyps or other bleeding lesions
▩ Gastroscopy / colonoscopy	▩ Looking for colonic polyps or other bleeding lesions; biopsies can also be taken in small / large intestine to check for signs of inflammatory bowel disease or coeliac disease

Diagnosis

Iron-deficiency anaemia

Clues to this diagnosis include a vegetarian diet and non-specific symptoms of lethargy, postural light-headedness and recent menorrhagia.

Lack of iron in the blood results in reduced ability for the body to produce haemoglobin.

Anaemia for investigation requires a large variety of investigations; however, each must be tailored depending on an accurate history and examination; iron studies are the gold standard in diagnosis of iron-deficiency anaemia.

Management

Lifestyle

▩ Diet: high iron intake (i.e. red meats, legumes, nuts)

Medical

▩ Oral iron supplements (over the counter): usually 3–6 months' therapy
▩ Iron infusion (ferrous carboxymaltose): IV infusion, 15–20 minutes
▩ Red cell transfusion: in settings where deficiency is secondary to blood loss or in patients with severe anaemia compromising end organ function (i.e. symptoms of anaemia, heart failure); with an iron infusion following the transfusion

In most cases, anaemia is an asymptomatic disease or only has minor symptoms – however in those with moderate to severe anaemia it can present with lethargy, dizziness, dyspnoea, palpitations, angina, jaundice, tachycardia and pallor

The causes for anaemia can be broken down into three major categories and can be managed differently:

▩ Blood loss:
  ● The simplest explanation for a decrease in haemoglobin is the loss of blood
  ● Secondary to trauma, ongoing gastro-intestinal bleeding, intra-operative blood loss, or in the above scenario from chronic blood loss due to likely uterine polyp

- Anaemia of unknown cause will always require investigation and screening to ensure there is no internal blood loss
- The gold standard for diagnosis of internal bleeding or checking for bleeding lesions is of course gastroscopy / colonoscopy and / or uteroscopy if uterine bleeding is suspected
- Biopsy of suspect lesions can also lead to a diagnosis of neoplastic processes, which can cause chronic anaemias

- Decreased red blood cell production:
  - Impaired production of red blood cells is generally broken down into either an inability to create cells in bone marrow (aplasia) or a lack of minerals required to mature red blood cells
  - The first pathology could be due to either a bone marrow red cell aplasia, aplastic anaemia (decreased production of all blood cells), or lack of erythropoietin due to renal failure
  - The lack of iron, B_{12}, and folic acid (haematinics) leads to an inability to mature erythroblasts – causing anaemia as well

- The treatment in these cases is to replete the haematinics and hence restore the ability for the body to complete maturation

- Increased red blood cell breakdown:
  - Certain haemoglobinopathies and enzyme deficiencies can lead to an increased breakdown of haemoglobin; in most cases these will present with jaundice, as bilirubin is a product of haemoglobin breakdown
  - An uncommon reason for this, but a good way of understanding the process, is that of antibody-mediated red cell breakdown; in the event of a wrong blood transfusion, antibodies will attack the foreign red blood cells, causing lysis and hence the release of bilirubin into serum; as such jaundice can be a sign of a transfusion reaction

Other differential diagnoses

- BPPV

Station 17 **Dyspepsia**

A 45-year-old man presents to the general surgery outpatient clinic referred by their GP with pain post eating and increased burning sensation in the chest.

Tasks

1 Take a history
2 Perform a physical examination

3 Describe appropriate investigations
4 Formulate a management plan

Differential diagnoses (VIITAMINC)

Vascular:
- Angina pectoris
- Acute coronary syndrome

Infective:
- Pneumonia
- Food poisoning

Inflammatory:
- Peptic ulcer disease
- Gastro-oesophageal reflux disease (GORD)
- Gastritis
- Cholelithiasis
- Pleurisy

Trauma

Autoimmune

Metabolic

Iatrogenic

Neoplastic:
- Gastric cancer

Congenital:
- Coeliac disease

Other:
- Gastroparesis
- Anxiety

Before starting

Establish rapport:
- Introduce yourself
- Obtain consent to take a history and examine the patient
- Exposure: when physical examination is required, it will require shirt / vest to be taken off

Confirm patient details:
- Name — *George Constantine*
- Age — *45 years*
- Occupation — *Businessman*

History

History of presenting complaint

- Onset: *started 1 week ago; initially intermittent, now constant*
- Location: *burning pain in the centre of the chest*
- Radiation: *no radiation*
- Exacerbating / relieving factors: *if hungry the pain worsens considerably; it gets better after eating a meal, but then it comes on a couple of hours after the meal*
- Nausea / vomiting: *occasional nausea when the pain begins, otherwise none*
- Appetite change: *no*
- Diet: *the occasional fatty meal, but likes Indian food*
- Weight loss: *no*
- Constitutional symptoms: *no fevers / rigors / chills*
- Haematemesis / coffee ground vomits: *none*
- Altered bowel habits: *no*
  - Haematochezia / melaena: *no*

Cardiovascular screen

- Pain worse on exertion: *no*

- Pain relieved on sitting up: *no*
- Shortness of breath on exertion: *no*
- Swelling in legs: *no*
- Syncopal episodes (fainting): *no*

Respiratory screen

- Cough: *no*
- Pain on inspiration: *no*

Past medical history and family history

- *Childhood asthma*
- *Father had heart attack at 75 years, mother had stroke at 70 years*

Drug history and allergies

- *No regular medications; but has been taking ibuprofen a lot more because the pain has worsened*
- *NKDA*

Social history

- Smoking history: *10 pack-years*
- Alcohol and drugs history: *one bottle of wine per day for the past 3 years; work has been very stressful; nil illicit drugs*

Examination

General inspection (ABCD-V)

- **A**ppearance: *patient looks comfortable while sitting up; no evident pain at this time*

- **B**ody habitus: *obese, BMI 31*
- **C**ognition: *patient is conscious and oriented*
- **D**evices / **D**rugs: *has a packet of ibuprofen with him, half empty*
- **V**itals: *BP 120/70mmHg, HR 70bpm and regular; other vital signs within normal range; afebrile*

Abdomen

- Inspection: *no surgical scars or visible pulsations*
- Palpation: *mild tenderness at the epigastric region of the abdomen; no evidence of abdominal aortic aneurysm (AAA); no evidence of portal hypertension*
- Percussion: *no ascites or organomegaly*
- Auscultation: *no bruits; bowel sounds present*

Chest:

- Inspection: *no surgical scars, deformities or visible pulsations; apex beat not visualised*
- Palpation: *apex beat not displaced, mid-clavicular 5th intercostal; no thrills or heaves are felt*
- Percussion: *no effusions notable; no dullness to percussion at posterior chest*
- Auscultation: *dual heart sounds with no murmurs; good air entry with symmetrical breath sounds; no added heart / airway sounds*

Investigations

BBMI-O: Bedside, **B**loods, **M**icrobiology, **I**maging and **O**ther

Investigation	Rationale
Bedside	
ECG	Looking for ECG changes associated with myocardial ischaemia, pericarditis or pulmonary embolism
Bloods	
FBC	Looking for infection and anaemia
CRP	Looking for infection
U&Es and creatinine	Looking for electrolyte imbalances, renal injury and raised urea (present in GI bleed)
Cardiac biomarkers	Looking for myocardial infarction

Investigation	Rationale
Microbiology	
Imaging	
CXR (PA and lateral views)	Looking for pneumoperitoneum, pulmonary infection and collapse; pleural effusion, cardiomegaly, mediastinal widening and rib fractures
CT neck / chest	Looking for signs of neck masses, oesophageal masses, upper chest masses
Other	
Gastroscopy	Looking for intra-oesophageal / gastric masses causing occlusion OR gastric / peptic ulcers

Diagnosis

Peptic ulcer disease (PUD)

The pattern of pain (worse when hungry and is relieved by food) and potential overuse of NSAIDs should raise suspicions of PUD.

The gold standard investigation to confirm PUD is gastroscopy.

Management

Lifestyle
- Smoking cessation
- Diet change – less spicy foods

Medical
- Anti-emetics and antacid medications (proton pump inhibitor (PPI) / H_2 antagonists) to decrease symptoms
- *Helicobacter pylori* treatment – triple therapy with antibiotics if proven.

Surgical
- Only necessary in the event of a bleeding or perforated peptic ulcer
- Bleeding peptic ulcers are treated either medically, or with gastroscopy and cautery
- Perforated PUD requires urgent surgery, with either laparoscopic or open approaches to identifying the ulcer, and patching of the affected area.

H. pylori is a helical-shaped rod, Gram-negative bacterium which is seen very commonly in patients with gastric ulcers, gastritis, duodenal ulcers, and has been linked to gastric cancer. The majority of patients who have it, however, are asymptomatic.

The diagnosis of *H. pylori* is made following the diagnosis of PUD. Urea breath testing is often undertaken as a non-invasive measure of testing for the bacterium; however, it can also be detected via biopsy during gastroscopy.

Medical therapy of the bacteria is undertaken via triple therapy treatment – the combination of omeprazole (PPI), and the dual antibiotics amoxicillin and clarithromycin. The therapy lasts for 1 week, with the PPI potentially lasting for 2 weeks or more. In some severe cases of *H. pylori*, bismuth citrate can also be added to the formula for more successful treatment.

Other differential diagnoses

- Cholelithiasis

Station 18 **Dysphagia**

A 66-year-old man presents to the upper gastrointestinal (GI) surgery outpatient clinic referred by his GP with difficulty on eating, and increased burning sensation in the chest, worsening over the past 6 months.

Tasks

1 Take a history
2 Perform a physical examination
3 Describe appropriate investigations
4 Formulate a management plan

Differential diagnoses (VIITAMINC)

Vascular:
- Aortic dissection

Infective:
- Pancreatitis
- Upper respiratory tract infection
- Pericarditis

Inflammatory:
- Oesophageal achalasia
- Barrett's oesophagus

Trauma:
- Oesophageal stricture
- Pneumothorax

Autoimmune

Metabolic

Iatrogenic

Neoplastic:
- Oesophageal cancer
- Lung cancer

Congenital

Other

Before starting

Establish rapport:
- Introduce yourself
- Obtain consent to take a history and examine the patient
- Exposure: when physical examination is required, it will require shirt / vest to be taken off

Confirm patient details:
- Name — *Simon Cavill*
- Age — *66 years*
- Occupation — *Construction worker, recently retired*

History

Dysphagia history / GI history
- Onset: *worsening over 6 months*
- Pain: *burning pain in nature, central chest, worse on eating*
- Difficulty eating: *feels in upper chest that food almost 'gets stuck'*
- Nausea / vomiting: *nausea worsening recently, no episodes of vomiting yet*
- Appetite change: *decreased appetite over past 3 months*
- Weight loss: *10kg weight loss over past 2 months, not actively dieting*

- Constitutional symptoms: *no fevers / rigors / chills*
- Haematemesis / coffee ground vomits: *one episode of vomiting, more red than usual*
- Altered bowel habits: *no*
- Haematochezia / melaena: *no*

Respiratory screen

- Coughing up any phlegm: *no*
- Pain on inspiration: *no*
- Haemoptysis: *no*

Cardiovascular screen

- Pain worse on exertion: *no*
- Pain relieved on sitting up: *no*
- Shortness of breath on exertion: *no*
- Swelling in legs: *no*
- Syncopal episodes (fainting): *no*

Past medical history and family history

- *Gastro-oesophageal reflux disease (GORD)*
- *Nil family history*

Drug history and allergies

- *Pantoprazole 40mg once daily, oral liquid antacid PRN*
- *NKDA*

Social history

- Smoking history: *20 pack-years*
- Alcohol and drugs history: *10 cans of beer per day, nil illicit drugs*

Examination

General inspection (ABCD-V)

- **A**ppearance: *patient looks comfortable while sitting up; no evident pain at this time*

- **B**ody habitus: *obese, BMI 33*
- **C**ognition: *patient is conscious and oriented*
- **D**evices / **D**rugs: *has a pack of pantoprazole on table*
- **V**itals: *BP 125/75mmHg, HR 80bpm and regular; other vital signs within normal range; afebrile*

Abdomen

- Inspection: *no surgical scars or visible pulsations*
- Palpation: *soft non-tender abdomen across all nine regions; no evidence of abdominal aortic aneurysm (AAA); no evidence of portal hypertension*
- Percussion: *no ascites or organomegaly*
- Auscultation: *no bruits; bowel sounds present*

Chest

- Inspection: *no surgical scars, deformities or visible pulsations; apex beat not visualised*
- Palpation: *apex beat not displaced, mid-clavicular 5th intercostal no thrills or heaves are felt*
- Percussion: *no effusions notable, no dullness to percussion at posterior chest*
- Auscultation: *dual heart sounds with no murmurs; good air entry with symmetrical breath sounds; no added heart / airway sounds*

Neck examination

- Inspection: *no evident masses, swelling*
- Palpation: *normal examination; no goitre noted; no masses noted*
- Percussion: *as above*
- Auscultation: *no carotid bruits, no added vasculature to be heard over thyroid area*

Investigations

BBMI-O: Bedside, **B**loods, **M**icrobiology, **I**maging and **O**ther

Investigation	Rationale
Bedside	
■ ECG	■ Looking for ECG changes associated with myocardial ischaemia, pericarditis or pulmonary embolism

Investigation	Rationale
Bloods	
▨ FBC	▨ Looking for infection and anaemia
▨ CRP	▨ Looking for infection
▨ U&Es and creatinine	▨ Looking for electrolyte imbalances and renal injury
▨ Cardiac biomarkers	▨ Looking for myocardial infarction
▨ Lipid profile	▨ Looking for hypercholesterolaemia
▨ TFTs	▨ Looking for hyper- / hypothyroidism
Microbiology	
Imaging	
▨ CXR (PA and lateral views)	▨ Looking for pulmonary infection and collapse; pleural effusion, cardiomegaly, mediastinal widening and rib fracture
▨ Echocardiogram	▨ Looking for ischaemic, pericardial and valvular heart disease
▨ Barium swallow	▨ Looking for narrowing of oesophagus and / or spasm of oesophagus
▨ CT neck / chest	▨ Looking for signs of neck masses, oesophageal masses, upper chest masses
▨ Gastroscopy	▨ Looking for intra-oesophageal / gastric masses causing occlusion OR gastric / peptic ulcers
Other	

Diagnosis

Oesophageal cancer

Insidious onset with unintentional weight loss and blood in vomit with a history of GORD, smoking and sedentary lifestyle increases suspicion for malignancy.

The gold standard investigation to confirm oesophageal cancer is gastroscopy.

Management

Medical

▨ Anti-emetics and antacid medications (proton pump inhibitors / H₂ antagonists) to decrease symptoms
▨ Chemotherapeutic / radiotherapeutic management – dependent on biopsy of the specimen and formal diagnosis

Surgical

▨ Surgical management will be dependent on the stage of oesophageal cancer, and dependent on biopsy of the specimen
▨ The optimal path for surgical resection of oesophageal cancer at this time is unknown – and is normally determined via thorough analysis of stage of cancer, and prognostic benefit

■ May require any of the following:
  ● Endoscopic resection of tumour alone
  ● Simple excision of tumour with mobilisation of stomach
  ● Oesophagectomy

In general

Stage 0 and 1 oesophageal cancer can be treated with surgical excision alone (endoscopic OR open).

Stage 2 and 3 oesophageal cancer will usually require preoperative chemotherapy prior to surgical excision, and postoperative radiotherapy.

Stage 4 oesophageal cancer would require chemoradiation prior to surgery, and consideration of further chemotherapy or radiotherapy postoperatively. Will likely require palliative care input due to progressive disease.

The majority of oesophageal cancers are adenocarcinoma, with less than 50% being of squamous cell carcinoma type. GI stromal tumours can also occur in the oesophagus and are usually benign.

Other differential diagnoses

■ Oesophageal achalasia
■ Barrett's oesophagus
■ Oesophageal stricture

Station 19 **Dyspnoea**

A 57-year-old man had a right knee replacement 5 days ago, and the nurse has asked for a medical review as he has become acutely short of breath.

Tasks

1 Take a history
2 Perform a physical examination
3 Describe appropriate investigations
4 Formulate a management plan

Differential diagnoses (VIITAMINC)

Vascular:
- Pulmonary embolism
- Acute pulmonary oedema
- Acute coronary syndrome

Infective:
- Pneumonia

Inflammatory:
- Asthma

Trauma

Autoimmune

Metabolic

Iatrogenic:
- Opiate overdose
- Sedating agents

Neoplastic

Congenital

Other:
- Atelectasis

Before starting

Establish rapport:
- Introduce yourself
- Obtain consent to take a history and examine the patient
- Exposure: when physical examination is required, it will require shirt / vest to be taken off

Confirm patient details:
- Name   *Eric White*
- Age   *57 years*
- Occupation   *Psychologist, currently practising*

History

History of presenting complaint
- Onset: *over the past few hours*
- Pain: *when breathing in, generalised across chest*

- How would you describe your breathing: *"difficult, I feel that I cannot take a full breath"*
- Cough: *initially when episode began, now subsided*
- Coughing up phlegm / blood: *at the start a small amount of blood; no further cough*
- Anything makes your breathing easier: *sitting up*
- Constitutional symptoms: *no fevers / rigors / chills*

Cardiovascular screen
- Is breathing worse on walking: *yes*
- Is pain relieved on sitting up: *no*
- Does pain radiate outside the chest: *no*
- Any swelling in legs: *right leg is more swollen and reddened than my left*
- Any syncopal episodes (fainting): *no*

Past medical history and family history
- *Nil significant past medical history*
- Family history: *sister has had a clot in her leg before spontaneously resolving*

Drug history and allergies

▨ *Not on anticoagulation*
▨ *Has been taking strong pain relief (opiates) infrequently*
▨ *NKDA*

Social history

▨ Smoking history: *5 pack-years*
▨ Alcohol and drugs history: *non-drinker, nil illicit drugs*

Examination

General inspection (ABCD-V)

▨ **A**ppearance: *patient looks in distress; laboured breathing*
▨ **B**ody habitus: *overweight, BMI 28*
▨ **C**ognition: *patient is conscious and oriented*
▨ **D**evices / **D**rugs: *has an oxygen mask next to him, but not wearing it; no inhalers*

▨ **V**itals: *BP 140/90mmHg, HR 110bpm and regular, RR 26 per minute; oxygen saturation at 92% on room air; afebrile*

Chest

▨ Inspection: *no surgical scars, deformities or visible pulsations; apex beat not visualised*
▨ Palpation: *apex beat not displaced, mid-clavicular 5th intercostal; no thrills or heaves are felt*
▨ Percussion: *no effusions notable; no dullness to percussion at posterior chest*
▨ Auscultation: *dual heart sounds with no murmurs; good air entry with symmetrical breath sounds; fine bi-basal crackles can be heard*

Lower limb examination

▨ Inspection: *right leg is swollen at the level of calf and erythematous compared with the left*
▨ Palpation: *tender right calf; hot to touch; peripheral leg pulses palpable and strong*
▨ Movement: *full range of movement noted*

Investigations

BBMI-O: Bedside, **B**loods, **M**icrobiology, **I**maging and **O**ther

Investigation	Rationale
Bedside	
▨ ECG	▨ Looking for ECG changes associated with myocardial ischaemia, pericarditis or pulmonary embolism (PE)
Bloods	
▨ FBC	▨ Looking for infection and anaemia
▨ CRP	▨ Looking for infection
▨ U&Es and creatinine	▨ Looking for electrolyte imbalances and renal injury
▨ Cardiac biomarkers	▨ Looking for myocardial infarction
▨ Lipid profile	▨ Looking for high cholesterol
▨ Thyroid function studies	▨ Looking for hyper- / hypothyroidism
▨ D-dimer	▨ Looking for increased risk of a clotting disorder

Investigation	Rationale
Microbiology	
Imaging	
▨ CXR (PA and lateral views)	▨ Looking for pulmonary infection and collapse; pleural effusion, and air bronchograms
▨ CT pulmonary angiogram	▨ Looking for evidence of pulmonary embolus in the bronchial segments
▨ VQ scan	▨ Looking for signs of ventilation / perfusion mismatch, potentially leading to a diagnosis of PE
▨ Right leg ultrasound	▨ Looking for deep vein thrombosis
Other	

Diagnosis

Pulmonary embolism (PE)

An acute episode of dyspnoea in a patient who has a red, hot, swollen calf with a history of recent surgery, is not on anticoagulation and has a family history of deep vein thrombosis (DVT) is very concerning, and investigations for PE must be performed.

The gold standard investigation to confirm PE is a CT pulmonary angiogram.

Discussion

PE is an acute life-threatening condition, which requires immediate diagnosis and treatment.

A blood clot that transmits its way to the lung and lodges in the airway is described as a pulmonary embolus. Its precursor is a DVT, which usually forms in the deep veins of the legs. The leg will thus present as swollen, tender and sometimes erythematous / hot to touch.

The risk of a patient to develop a pulmonary embolus can be classified according to the Wells' criteria. The criteria are as follows:

Wells' criteria

Criterion	Yes	No
Clinical signs of deep vein thrombosis?	+3	+0
Is PE the number one diagnosis or equally likely?	+3	+0
Is the heart rate >100bpm?	+1.5	+0
Immobilisation at least 3 days OR surgery in previous 4 weeks?	+1.5	+0

Criterion	Yes	No
Previously, objectively diagnosed PE?	+1.5	+0
Haemoptysis?	+1	+0
Malignancy with treatment within the past 6 months or palliative patient?	+1	+0

If ≤4: PE unlikely, can consider a D-dimer

If ≥4.5: PE likely, should consider CT pulmonary angiogram

Management

Medical

- Supportive measures such as high-flow oxygen should be immediately administered
- The patient should be considered for cardiac monitoring and intensive care support
- Therapeutic anticoagulation can then be used in the form of low molecular weight heparin, or a direct oral anticoagulant
- Thrombolysis is an established method of treatment for massive pulmonary embolus

Surgical

- Surgical management is rarely performed and would be considered outside the scope of usually suggested management at this level of training
- Pulmonary embolectomy is currently a rare procedure with high mortality rates; it is only performed in the context of a massive or sub-massive PE

Other differential diagnoses

- Atelectasis

Station 20 **Earache**

A 16-year-old boy presents to his GP with a 2-day history of right ear pain.

Tasks

1 Take a history

2 Perform a physical examination

3 Describe appropriate investigations

4 Formulate a management plan

Differential diagnoses

Otolaryngological (ear):

■ Acute otitis media

■ Otitis externa

■ Labyrinthitis

■ Foreign body

■ Herpes zoster infection

Otolaryngological (other):

■ Tonsillitis

■ Sinusitis

■ Pharyngitis

■ Trigeminal neuralgia

Before starting

Establish rapport:

■ Introduce yourself

■ Obtain consent to take a history and examine the patient

■ Exposure – as appropriate; will not need exposure unless performing respiratory exam as addendum

Confirm patient details:

■ Name	*Dawid Michalak*
■ Age	*16 years*
■ Occupation	*Student*

History

History of presenting complaint

■ Onset: *over the past 2 days*

■ Site: *in the right ear*

■ Describe the pain: *constant throbbing, a dull pain*

■ Radiation: *no*

■ Exacerbating / relieving factors: *taking paracetamol seems to help; nothing else*

■ Associated symptoms: *sore throat for a few days before it started; no headaches*

■ Change in hearing: *a little bit dull in the right ear*

■ Discharge from the ear: *occasional yellow discharge started yesterday*

■ Dizziness: *no*

■ Rash: *no*

■ Previous episodes: *this is the fourth time in the past month; usually takes antibiotics and it goes away*

■ Constitutional symptoms: *fevers since yesterday*

Past medical history and family history

■ *Nil significant past medical history*

■ *Nil family history*

Drug history and allergies

■ *No regular medications; paracetamol PRN*

■ *NKDA*

Social history

■ Smoking history: *non-smoker*

■ Alcohol history: *non-drinker*

Examination

General inspection (ABCD-V)

■ **A**ppearance: *patient looks comfortable*

■ **B**ody habitus: *normal, BMI 22*

■ **C**ognition: *the patient is conscious and oriented*

■ **D**evices / **D**rugs: *nil*
■ **V**itals: *BP 110/80mmHg, HR 65bpm and regular; febrile at 37.8°C*

ENT examination

■ Inspection:
- Ear: *small amount of discharge coming out of the right ear, purulent in nature; no cellulitis, no masses*
- Nose: *normal inspection, no septal deviation, no discharge from nose*
- Throat: *reddened back of throat, no evident tonsillitis*
■ Palpation:
- Ear: *no mastoid tenderness; skin not hot to touch*
- Nose: *no evident deformity; no fractures*

■ Otoscopy:
- Right middle ear: *tympanum is dull / foggy; small hole evident with discharging liquid*

Neck examination

■ Submental lymph nodes: *normal*
■ Submandibular lymph nodes: *enlarged right node compared to left, tender to palpation*
■ Anterior chain lymph nodes: *normal*
■ Posterior chain lymph nodes: *normal*
■ Occipital lymph nodes: *normal*

Cranial nerve examination

■ *All cranial nerves from I to XII are considered normal for this examination; otherwise no evident nerve palsy or abnormalities*

Investigations

BBMI-O: Bedside, **B**loods, **M**icrobiology, **I**maging and **O**ther

Investigation	Rationale
Bedside	
Bloods	
■ FBC	■ Looking for infection and anaemia
■ CRP	■ Looking for infection / inflammation
■ U&Es and creatinine	■ Looking for electrolyte imbalances and renal injury
Microbiology	
■ Swab for MCS	■ Looking for bacterial growth in ear discharge
Imaging	
■ CT / MRI head / neck	■ Looking for any internal collections, masses, or nerve lesions that may cause pain; further looking for lymphadenopathy
Other	
■ Audiometry	■ Looking for conductive hearing loss pre-treatment and post-treatment associated with middle / inner ear infection

Diagnosis

Acute otitis media

Ear pain with discharge that is responsive to antibiotics is most likely a bacterial infection – the location of infection behind the tympanic membrane is suggestive of otitis media.

Management

Treatment for acute otitis media is rarely surgical; however, recurrent cases or chronic cases can benefit from surgical management. Otherwise, treatment is as described below.

Medical

- Supportive measures such as analgesia, and antipyrexials such as paracetamol and ibuprofen, can assist in the initial conservative management of otitis media
- Antibiotic therapy can be indicated in severe cases, those with proven bacterial growth on swab, or those not responding to conservative measures; first-line management involves oral amoxicillin or amoxicillin / clavulanate in severe cases
- Topical therapies such as ciprofloxacin eardrops can also be considered; however, evidence to suggest a superior outcome is limited

Surgical

- Tympanostomy tube (or 'grommet'): for recurrent or chronic otitis media only; the surgical treatment of choice is usually used in younger children, who have otitis media for between 1 and 3 months; it is creation of a small hole in the tympanic membrane to allow for the passage of discharge, to ensure no build-up of discharge and reduce the risk of perforation
- The criterion for inserting a tympanostomy tube is strict; however, it is a commonplace procedure in the paediatric population; the insertion of a tympanostomy does NOT prevent all occurrences of otitis media; hence careful re-examination should occur should further recurrences appear

Not all otitis media has discharge (i.e. suppurative otitis media). With the majority of cases being non-suppurative in nature, it is therefore important that careful examination takes place and that a review of all otolaryngology systems is examined. Otitis media commonly occurs post upper respiratory tract infection and the treatment of this pathology may lead to the treatment of the otitis. A good view of the ear must be obtained to check for the presence of foreign bodies which can be removed under otoscopy; difficult cases can be referred to ENT surgeons for further management.

Other differential diagnoses

- Otitis externa

Station 21 **Facial ulcer**

A 50-year-old farmer has come to see you in your GP practice wanting an opinion on a facial lesion that has been there for the past year but has started bleeding over the last few months.

Tasks

1 Take a history
2 Perform a targeted examination

3 Describe appropriate investigations
4 Formulate a management plan

Differential diagnoses (VIITAMINC)

Vascular

Infective:
- Herpes simplex virus
- Abscess

Inflammatory:
- Insect bites
- Warts
- Solar keratosis
- Acne

Trauma

Autoimmune

Metabolic

Iatrogenic

Neoplastic:
- Basal cell carcinoma
- Squamous cell carcinoma
- Melanoma
- Keratoacanthoma

Congenital

Other:
- Sebaceous cyst

Before starting

Establish rapport:
- Introduce yourself
- Obtain consent to take a history and examine the patient
- Exposure: as appropriate; patient will not need exposure unless investigating another system as addendum

Confirm patient details:
- Name — *John Downer*
- Age — *50 years*
- Occupation — *Farmer*

History

History of presenting complaint

- Pain: *no*

- Onset: *initially noticed 2 years ago, though in the last 3 months it has grown and started to bleed*
- Location: *the lesion is on the nose; other spots which were similar to how it looked initially are located at the ears, back of the neck and arms*
- Itch: *yes*
- Discharge: *blood*
- Exacerbating / relieving factors: *no*
- Fevers / sweats / chills: *no*
- Lethargy / weight loss: *otherwise well, no lethargy or weight loss noticed*

Past medical history and family history

- *Osteoarthritis and hypertension*
- *Previous melanoma excision on the left arm 5 years ago*
- *Father had many skin lesions excised over his lifetime; mother had osteoarthritis*

Drug history and allergies

- Panadol PRN, ramipril
- NKDA

Social history

- Smoking history: non-smoker
- Alcohol and drugs history: non-drinker, nil illicit drugs
- Works as farmer, has direct sun exposure

Examination

General inspection (ABCD-V)

- **A**ppearance: patient has sunburnt skin throughout with obvious 'tan lines' where clothed
- **B**ody habitus: normal, BMI 24

- **C**ognition: patient is oriented
- **D**evices / Drugs: nil
- **V**itals: BP 120/80mmHg, HR 85bpm irregularly irregular, RR 16 per minute; oxygen saturation at 100% on room air; temperature 37.4°C

Skin examination

- Location: lesion is adjacent to the nares of the right nostril
- Colour and morphology: it is a red pearly colour with a raised edge / nodular appearance with telangiectasia and a central region of ulceration and bleeding
- Size: it is approximately 6mm
- Surrounding skin: normal
- Lymph nodes: no lymphadenopathy

Investigations

BBMI-O: Bedside, **B**loods, **M**icrobiology, **I**maging and **O**ther

Investigation	Rationale
Bedside	
Bloods	
FBC	Looking for infection and anaemia
U&Es and creatinine	Looking for electrolyte imbalances and renal injury
ESR	Looking for potential for rheumatoid disease
Rheumatoid factor	Looking for potential for rheumatoid disease
Viral serologies e.g. HSV, CMV, HIV	To rule out viral rashes
Microbiology	
Wound MCS	If concerns of infection, one may do a wound MCS
Imaging	
CT chest, abdomen, pelvis	If suspecting a metastatic disease process especially like melanoma; however, in this case this would be unlikely
Other	
Patch testing	Not required here, but if suspected allergic type reaction may consider
Excisional biopsy	Looking for malignancy

Diagnosis

Basal cell carcinoma (BCC)

A red, pearly skin lesion with central ulceration and bleeding and a raised edge is morphology that is suspicious of BCC.

The gold standard for diagnosis of BCC is an excisional biopsy.

Management

Medical

- For superficial small lesions not on face: 5-fluorouracil / imiquimod cream may be considered
- Biopsy or excision initially is recommended to get a diagnosis

Surgical

- Excisional biopsy with a 3–5mm margin is the most appropriate for this lesion
- Mohs micrographic surgery

Other

- Radiotherapy in those unfit for surgery
- Photodynamic therapy for superficial lesions
- Cryotherapy for superficial lesions away from face / neck

Other differential diagnoses

- Amelanotic melanoma
- Seborrhoeic keratosis
- Fibrous papule
- Keratoacanthoma
- Squamous cell skin carcinoma

Useful terminology

Macule: <1cm of altered skin colour	**Patch:** >1cm of altered skin colour	**Papule:** palpable mass on skin <0.5cm	**Nodule:** palpable mass on skin >0.5cm
Plaque: flat-topped palpable mass >1cm	**Maculopapule:** raised and discoloured lesion	**Wheal:** raised lesion secondary to dermal oedema that is pale and compressible	**Vesicle:** blister <0.5cm
Bulla: vesicle >0.5cm	**Pustule:** purulent collection in skin <1cm	**Abscess:** purulent collection in skin >1cm	**Purpura:** purpuric lesion 0.3–10cm
Ecchymosis: purpuric lesion >10cm	**Petechiae:** purpuric lesion <3mm	**Ulcer:** circumscribed deep defect with loss of epidermis and part or all of the dermis	

Station 22 **Facial weakness**

An 80-year-old woman is brought in by ambulance to the emergency department with new left facial droop and left-sided weakness noted by her granddaughter.

Tasks

1 Take a history
2 Perform a targeted examination

3 Describe appropriate investigations
4 Formulate a management plan

Differential diagnoses

- Stroke
- Transient ischaemic attack
- Bell's palsy
- Intracranial haemorrhage
- Epidural haematoma

- Central nervous system vasculitis
- Reversible cerebral vasoconstriction syndrome
- Cerebral tumour
- Seizures with Todd's paralysis

Before starting

Establish rapport:
- Introduce yourself
- Obtain consent to take a history and examine the patient
- Exposure: when physical examination is required, inform the patient that the area you will examine is exposed appropriately

Confirm patient details:
- Name   *Beryl Stone*
- Age   *80 years*
- Occupation   *Retired*

History

The patient is confused, and history is taken from daughter:
- Time of onset: *first noticed this morning on waking, though it has been getting worse over the day; the weakness is on the left side of her body: face, arm and leg*
- Shaking / biting of tongue / unusual sensations / urinary or bowel incontinence: *no*
- Confusion: *yes*
- Recent mobility issues / falls history: *she has been having an increased number of falls over*

the last 6 months, one every week, the last being last night; she just states that she becomes a 'bit unsteady'
- Blood thinners: *no*
- Fevers / neck stiffness / photophobia / recent flu-like symptoms / sick contacts: *no*
- Last meal: *this morning at 8am*

Pain history (SOCRATES)
- **S**ite: *headache*
- **O**nset: *"not too sure, but did have a fall when she went to the toilet last night; I think she hit her head then"*
- **C**haracter: *constant frontal ache in the front of head*
- **R**adiation: *nil*
- **A**ssociation: *unsure*
- **T**ime: *she has had a lot of falls recently*
- **E**xacerbating / relieving factors: *nil*
- **S**everity: *it must be 7–8/10*

Past medical history and family history
- *Osteoarthritis, type 2 diabetes mellitus, congestive heart failure, hypertension*
- *Nil family history*

Drug history and allergies
- *NSAIDs, metformin, furosemide, perindopril*
- *NKDA*

Social history

▨ Smoking history: *non-smoker*
▨ Alcohol and drugs history: *non-drinker,
   nil illicit drugs*
▨ *Usually independent at home by herself, though
   over last few months has been declining*

Examination

General inspection (ABCD-V)

▨ **A**ppearance: *patient is visibly confused and
   agitated*
▨ **B**ody habitus: *normal, BMI 24*
▨ **C**ognition: *patient is oriented*
▨ **D**evices / **D**rugs: *nil*
▨ **V**itals: *BP 120/80mmHg, HR 85bpm irregularly
   irregular, RR 16 per minute; oxygen saturation at
   100% on room air; temperature 37.4°C*

Neurological examination

Glasgow Coma Score (GCS) 13 – E3V4M6
▨ Cranial nerve examination:
   • *CN II pupils 3mm bilaterally reactive;
     normal fields and acuity*

• *CN III, IV, VI full range of motion;
  no nystagmus / ophthalmoplegia*
• *CN V motor and sensory function intact*
• *CN VII obvious left facial droop, with
  lower face muscular weakness*
• *CN VIII, IX, X not performed*
• *CN XI full power sternocleidomastoid and
  trapezius*
• *CN XII not deviated; upper limb (UL) and
  lower limb (LL) examination*
▨ Tone: *slightly increased on the left UL / LL normal*
▨ *Pronator drift on the left UL; no clonus on the LL*
▨ *Power of the left upper limb (UL) is 4/5 in all
  muscle groups. Power is 5/5 in the right UL and
  both LL (lower limbs)*
▨ Reflexes: *slightly more brisk on the left UL,
  otherwise normal*
▨ Sensation: *intact throughout*
▨ Proprioception: *intact*
▨ Coordination: *intact but more difficulty with
  left UL*

Investigations

BBMI-O: Bedside, **B**loods, **M**icrobiology, **I**maging and **O**ther

Investigation	Rationale
Bedside	
▨ ECG	▨ Looking for arrhythmia
Bloods	
▨ FBC	▨ Looking for inflammation, platelets, anaemia
▨ U&Es and creatinine	▨ Looking for electrolyte imbalances and renal injury
▨ Coagulation studies	▨ Looking for coagulation profile in case patient is for an operation
▨ Blood, group and hold	▨ Patient may be for an operation
Microbiology	

Investigation	Rationale
Imaging	
CT brain ± contrast ± perfusion	If suspecting a lesion causing these symptoms, a contrast CT would be reasonable
	If suspecting a stroke, a CT perfusion would be the test of choice; in this case, a CT brain non-contrast with bony windows for skull should be carried out looking for acute blood which is hyperdense on CT (chronic blood is hypodense)
Other	

Diagnosis

Subdural haematoma

A history of recent falls and subacute time course is more suggestive of a subdural haematoma.

The gold standard to diagnose a subdural haematoma is a CT brain.

Management

Medical / conservative

- If the patient is having seizures they should be started on anti-epileptics
- Reverse coagulopathy
- Head of bed 30 degrees
- Mannitol and indwelling catheter if signs of raised intracranial pressure (ICP)
- Conservative management with repeat CT brain may be a reasonable option in those unfit for surgery or those with small subdural haematomas

Surgical

- Evacuation of subdural haematoma via burr holes or craniotomy.
- In cases with evidence of raised ICP, or progressively worsening symptoms such as seizures / reduced GCS

Other differential diagnoses

- Epidural haematoma
- Ischaemic stroke
- Bell's palsy

Station 23 **Fever in a returned traveller**

A 21-year-old student returned from a trip to India over a month ago, and is now presenting with abdominal pain and fevers.

Tasks

1 Take a history
2 Perform a targeted examination

3 Describe appropriate investigations
4 Name three differential diagnoses

Differential diagnoses (VIITAMINC)

Vascular:
- Pulmonary embolism

Infective:
- Bacterial:
  - Tuberculosis
  - Brucellosis
  - Typhoid
  - Leptospirosis
  - Q fever
  - Salmonella
  - Legionnaires' disease
- Viral:
  - Cytomegalovirus
  - Epstein–Barr virus
  - Varicella zoster
  - HIV
  - Dengue
  - Influenza
  - Middle East respiratory syndrome
  - Hepatitis
- Parasitic:
  - Malaria
  - Toxoplasmosis

- Schistosomiasis
- Giardia
- Pneumonia – bacterial / viral / fungal
- Cholangitis
- Cholecystitis
- Liver abscess

Inflammatory:
- Gastritis
- Choledocholithiasis
- Biliary colic

Trauma:
- Pneumothorax

Autoimmune

Metabolic

Iatrogenic

Neoplastic

Congenital

Other

Before starting

Establish rapport:
- Introduce yourself
- Obtain consent to take a history and examine the patient

- Expose the patient: when physical examination is required inform the patient that the area you will examine is exposed appropriately

Confirm patient details:
- Name   *John Tucker*
- Age   *21 years*
- Occupation   *Student*

History

Pain history (SOCRATES)

- **S**ite: *tummy is really sore; mainly over the right upper abdomen*
- **O**nset: *progressively worsened over the past week*
- **C**haracter: *dull pain*
- **R**adiation: *radiates to shoulder*
- **A**ssociation: *some nausea, vomiting and loss of appetite*
- **T**ime: *it seems to be there all the time*
- **E**xacerbating / relieving factors: *deep breathing seems to make it worse*
- **S**everity: *7/10*

Travel history (CHOCOLATES)

- **C**ontacts: *no*
- **H**ousing: *communal*
- **O**ccupation: *student*
- **C**ountry of origin: *Australia*
- **O**ther (immunisations, IV drug use, immunosuppression, other sick contacts): *no*
- **L**eisure activities carried out: *sightseeing in the north and swimming at the beaches in the south of India*
- **A**nimal exposures: *no*
- **T**ravel and travel prophylaxis: *recent return from India, did not get any recommended travel vaccinations*
- **E**ating and drinking: *was relatively careful when travelling, though there were a few times where food was prepared in a questionable setting*
- **S**exual contact: *yes, multiple partners, though uses protection*

Other

- General health: *well otherwise*
- Any weight loss: *yes*
- Fatigue: *yes*
- Pattern of fevers: *occasionally will have a fever*
- Shortness of breath / chest pain / palpitations: *no*

- Change in bowel habits: *yes, had a bout of diarrhoea while in India, still ongoing though slightly improved*
- Change of skin colour: *mother had commented that skin was looking a little yellow*

Past medical history and family history

- *Nil significant past medical history*
- *Grandfather had a heart attack at 80 years*

Drug history and allergies

- *Nil*
- *NKDA*

Social history

- Smoking history: *5 pack-years*
- Alcohol and drugs history: *social drinker, nil illicit drugs*
- Occupation: *student*

Examination

General inspection (ABCD-V)

- **A**ppearance: *patient is uncomfortable, visibly jaundiced*
- **B**ody habitus: *normal, BMI 21*
- **C**ognition: *patient is oriented*
- **D**evices / **D**rugs: *nil aids*
- **V**itals: *BP 125/91mmHg, HR 110bpm regular, RR 18 per minute; oxygen saturation at 98% on room air; temperature 38.1°C*

Abdominal examination

- Inspection: *nil bruising or erythema, nil caput medusae or spider naevi*
- Palpation: *abdomen is soft with right upper quadrant tenderness; Murphy negative; fullness in the right upper quadrant; nil splenomegaly*
- Percussion: *nil signs of peritonism*
- Auscultation: *normal bowel sounds*

Investigations

BBMI-O: Bedside, **B**loods, **M**icrobiology, **I**maging and **O**ther

Investigation	Rationale
Bedside	
Bloods	
▪ FBC	▪ Looking for infection and anaemia
▪ U&Es and creatinine	▪ Looking for electrolyte imbalances and renal injury
▪ LFTs	▪ May have deranged LFTs especially alkaline phosphatase
▪ Blood cultures	▪ As part of septic screen – to identify the causative organism
▪ Coagulation studies	▪ Looking for coagulation profile as the patient may be for an intervention
▪ Blood sugar level and HbA1c	▪ Looking for diabetes mellitus and its potential complications
▪ Entamoeba antibody test	▪ Can be considered if it is thought that *Entamoeba* spp. is the cause
Microbiology	
▪ Sputum MCS	▪ To isolate a causative organism
▪ Stool MCS	
▪ Fluid aspirate	
Imaging	
▪ CT abdomen and pelvis	▪ May see hypodense liver lesions; some may show rim enhancement; some may show gas which suggests pyogenic abscess
▪ US liver	▪ Echoic lesions seen; also can be used as a guide to drain lesion
▪ CXR	▪ As part of a septic screen
Other	

Diagnosis

Liver abscess

The gold standard to diagnose liver abscess is a CT abdomen.

Management

Medical

- IV fluids and resuscitation (if unstable)
- IV antibiotics e.g. ceftriaxone and metronidazole if pyogenic OR metronidazole / tinidazole if amoebic; analgesia

Surgical

- If a large abscess or failed medical treatment – US-guided drainage (usually if >5cm, left lobe lesions, risk of rupture)

Other differential diagnoses

- Cholangitis
- Cholecystitis
- Hepatocellular carcinoma
- Viral hepatitis

Station 24 **Finger pain**

A 75-year-old retired construction worker has come to the surgical outpatient clinic with 6 months of severe right finger pain.

Tasks

1 Take a history and examination
2 Perform a targeted examination

3 Describe appropriate investigations
4 Formulate a management plan

Differential diagnoses (VIITAMINC)

Vascular

Infective

Inflammatory:
- Carpal tunnel syndrome
- Ulnar nerve syndrome
- Cervical spine degeneration / disease
- Peripheral neuropathy
- Tenosynovitis
- Osteoarthritis
- Inflammatory arthritis – psoriatic arthritis, rheumatoid arthritis

Trauma:
- Tendon rupture

- Fracture
- Dislocation
- Sprain

Autoimmune

Metabolic:
- Acromegaly
- Hypothyroidism

Iatrogenic

Neoplastic

Congenital

Other

Before starting

Establish rapport:
- Introduce yourself
- Obtain consent to take a history and examine the patient
- Expose the patient: when physical examination is required, inform the patient that the area you will examine is exposed appropriately

Confirm patient details:
- Name   *Mark Bentham*
- Age   *75 years*
- Occupation   *Retired*

History

Pain history (SOCRATES)

- **S**ite: *right index finger and thumb very painful*

- **O**nset: *progressively worsened over the past 2 years*
- **C**haracter: *stiffness and discomfort all the time, more tender / sharp pain at the end of the day*
- **R**adiation: *no*
- **A**ssociation: *none known, though definitely worse with more use of the hand*
- **T**ime: *better in the morning, worsens as the day goes on*
- **E**xacerbating / relieving factors: *excessive use of the fingers makes it worse, paracetamol improves the pain a little but not so much lately*
- **S**everity: *baseline 3–4/10, lately an 8/10*

Neurological history

- Recent trauma to neck, hand or arm: *no*
- Weakness / loss of power: *yes, due to pain and stiffness*
- Paraesthesia / numbness: *no*

- Bladder or bowel incontinence: *no*
- Issues with walking: *no*

Musculoskeletal history

- Painful or stiff joints: *yes, as above*
- Red or swollen joints: *some days the thumb and index finger swell at the end of the day*
- Skin rash: *no*
- Back or neck pain: *no*
- Loss of motion: *yes, due to pain and stiffness*
- Loss of function: *no*
- Joint instability: *no*
- Crepitations / scraping of joints on movement: *yes, fingers feel as though they are grinding together*

Other

- *Well otherwise*
- Weight gain: *no*
- Fatigue: *no*
- Ring tighter / shoe size increase: *no*

Past medical history and family history

- *Type 2 diabetes mellitus (T2DM), hypertension, hypercholesterolaemia*
- *Father had T2DM and stroke at 85 years, mother had osteoarthritis in multiple joints*

Drug history and allergies

- *Regular medications include atorvastatin, captopril and metformin*
- *NKDA*

Social history

- Smoking history: *non-smoker*
- Alcohol and drugs history: *non-drinker, nil illicit drugs*
- Occupation: *retired, previous construction worker*
- House setting: *at home with wife, independent of all activities of daily living, though finding it harder lately with this pain*

Examination

General inspection (ABCD-V)

- **A**ppearance: *patient is comfortable*
- **B**ody habitus: *normal, BMI 24*
- **C**ognition: *patient is oriented*

- **D**evices / **D**rugs: *nil aids*
- **V**itals: *all within normal limits*

Upper limb neurological examination

- Inspection of upper limb / hand: *no scars or deformities*
- Tone: *normal bilaterally*
- Power: *normal 5/5 for the left hand, 4+/5 for right hand, limited ability to test finger flexion / extension due to pain*
- Reflexes: *normal biceps, triceps, brachioradialis; Hoffman negative*
- Coordination: *normal*
- Sensation: *normal bilaterally*
- Tinel's test over the flexor retinaculum / Phalen's test: *negative*
- Spurling test: *negative*

Rheumatological hand examination

- Inspection:
  - Erythema, rash and swelling: *thumb and index finger on the right hand appear swollen, no rash / erythema or altered skin colour*
  - Intrinsic muscle appearance: *no wasting*
  - Heberden's (distal interphalangeal, DIP) and Bouchard's (proximal interphalangeal, PIP) nodes: *present on index, middle and ring fingers bilaterally*
  - Swan neck deformity, boutonniere deformity, Z deformity: *no*
  - Ulnar deviation: *no*
  - Dactylitis (sausage digits): *no*
  - Gouty tophi: *no*
  - Nails: *no changes*
- Palpation:
  - Joint lines: *tenderness on palpation over the right thumb and index finger*
  - Joint effusion / bogginess: *no*
  - Ulnar styloid: *no tenderness*
  - Stress tenderness (at metacarpophalangeal (MCP) joint and wrist): *negative*
- Movement:
  - Wrist: *normal bilaterally*
  - MCP: *normal bilaterally*
  - PIP and DIP: *reduced flexion / extension in the 2nd to 4th digits bilaterally, especially the*

thumb and index finger on the right due to pain; *abduction / adduction normal bilaterally*
- Grip strength: *reduced bilaterally, right worse than left*

- Functional movements (undo a button, key grip, pen grip): *able to perform all but with some difficulty*

Investigations

BBMI-O: Bedside, **B**loods, **M**icrobiology, **I**maging and **O**ther

Investigation	Rationale
Bedside	
Bloods	
FBC	Looking for anaemia and infection
CRP, ESR	Looking for inflammation
±Glucose level and HbA1c	Looking for diabetes mellitus and its potential complications of peripheral neuropathy
±IGF1, GH suppression test, TSH, T_3/T_4, RF, anti-CCP, ANA	Can be considered if it is thought that other pathologies are the underlying cause of carpal tunnel syndrome
Rheumatoid factor	Looking for rheumatoid arthritis
Uric acid	Looking for gout
Microbiology	
Imaging	
X-ray of bilateral hands	Looking for arthritic changes: • Loss of joint space • Osteophytes • Subchondral sclerosis • Subchondral cysts
MRI spine	If suspecting spinal cord pathology, especially if unsure if cervical spine pathology is causing symptoms, it would be reasonable to order an MRI spine
Other	
Nerve conduction studies	If concerned the pain is neuropathic in nature (e.g. carpal tunnel syndrome, ulnar nerve syndrome)
Joint aspiration	For MCS and cell count, to differentiate between inflammatory and septic joints; for diagnosis of gout, calcium urate is positive with needle-shaped crystals; for the diagnosis of pseudogout, positive birefringence is present

Diagnosis

Osteoarthritis

A relatively benign history and insidious onset with Heberden's and Bouchard's nodes on examination is highly suggestive of osteoarthritis.

Management

Lifestyle

- Regular exercise and strengthening exercises
- Physiotherapy input
- Occupational therapy input for activities of daily life assistance

Medical

- Paracetamol: for mild–moderate pain, as required and as a baseline in flares
- NSAID:
  - Oral (e.g. celecoxib): should be used concomitantly with proton pump inhibitor
  - Topical (e.g. diclofenac)
- Intra-articular corticosteroid injections: for short-term relief in acute exacerbations with joint effusions and local inflammation
- Opioids (e.g. oxycodone): for short-term use in acute exacerbations
- Duloxetine: chronic pain management

Surgical

- Procedures available: ulnar head replacement, MCP joint replacement / fusion, pisiform excision, wrist fusion (arthrodesis), PIP replacement

Other differential diagnoses

- Rheumatoid arthritis
- Pseudogout
- Psoriatic arthritis

Station 25 **Foot pain**

A 75-year-old retiree presents to the emergency department with several hours of worsening left foot pain.

Tasks

1 Take a history and examination
2 Perform a targeted examination
3 Describe appropriate investigations
4 Formulate a management plan

Differential diagnoses (VIITAMINC)

Vascular:
- Acute limb ischaemia
- Chronic limb ischaemia
- Raynaud's phenomenon

Infective

Inflammatory:
- Tarsal tunnel syndrome
- Lumbar spine pathologies
- Peripheral neuropathy with dyaesthesiae
- Gout
- Osteoarthritis
- Plantar fasciitis
- Inflammatory arthritis – psoriatic arthritis, rheumatoid arthritis

- Morton's neuroma

Trauma:
- Tendon rupture
- Fracture
- Dislocation
- Sprain

Autoimmune

Metabolic

Iatrogenic

Neoplastic

Congenital

Other

Before starting

Establish rapport:
- Introduce yourself
- Obtain consent to take a history and examine the patient
- Exposure: when physical examination is required, inform the patient that the area you will examine is exposed appropriately

Confirm patient details:
- Name   *Alex Paphides*
- Age   *75 years*
- Occupation   *Retired mechanic*

History

Pain history (SOCRATES)
- **S**ite: *left foot is painful*
- **O**nset: *progressively worsened over the past 3 hours*
- **C**haracter: *ache, burning*
- **R**adiation: *some pain in the calf*
- **A**ssociation: *foot also is numb now; pain worse with standing*
- **T**ime: *sudden onset*
- **E**xacerbating / relieving factors: *tried some oxycodone which helped a little*
- **S**everity: *9/10*

Take a focused history

- Recent trauma: *no*
- Pins and needles or numbness: *no*
- Pain in the back of legs / calves when walking: *no*
- Bladder or bowel incontinence: *no*
- Gait disturbance: *no*
- Fevers, sweats, chills: *no*

Past medical history and family history

- *Atrial fibrillation (AF), type 2 diabetes mellitus, acute myocardial infarction, hypertension, hypercholesterolaemia*
- *Nil family history*

Drug history and allergies

- *Warfarin, metformin, clopidogrel, rosuvastatin, amlodipine, enalapril*

Social history

- Smoking history: *35 pack-years*
- Alcohol and drugs history: *3 standard alcohol units per day, nil illicit drugs*
- Recently retired; lives sedentary lifestyle at home

Examination

General inspection (ABCD-V)

- **A**ppearance: *patient is clearly in pain and in discomfort*
- **B**ody habitus: *obese, BMI 31*
- **C**ognition: *patient is oriented*
- **D**evices / **D**rugs: *nil aids*
- **V**itals: *within normal limits*

Lower limb examination

- Inspection:
  - Left: *no scars or deformities; pallor of lower leg especially prominent from below knee; feels cold*
  - Right: *normal*
- Palpation:
  - *Calves soft bilaterally*
  - Left: *pulses absent posterior tibialis, dorsal pedis and popliteal pulses; the area where popliteal artery is feels swollen; capillary refill absent*
  - Right: *normal*
  - *Femoral arterial pulses present bilaterally*
- Buerger's B test: *negative*
- *Normal power 5/5 throughout lower limb except the movement of toes, ankle eversion, inversion, plantar flexion and dorsiflexion four-fifths on the left; right normal*
- *Sensation loss more prominent in feet*
- Ankle Doppler pressure: *ankle-brachial index (ABI) on left lower limb 0.3; Doppler signal from femoral artery but not from popliteal and below*

Abdominal examination

- *Unremarkable, nil expansile pulsations from abdominal aorta*

Investigations

BBMI-O: Bedside, **B**loods, **M**icrobiology, **I**maging and **O**ther

Investigation	Rationale
Bedside	
Ankle-brachial index	As carried out in the examination
ECG	May diagnose new AF
Bloods	
FBC	Baseline level also to assess if any issues predisposing to thrombosis
U&Es and creatinine	Baseline level and may have elevated potassium with dying tissue
Coagulation studies	Looking for coagulation profile as patient is likely for an operation / heparin infusion

Investigation	Rationale
±Blood glucose level and HbA1c	Looking for diabetes mellitus and its potential complications of peripheral neuropathy
Arterial blood gases	To assess for acidosis
Group and hold	Anyone who potentially is undergoing surgery especially with high risk of bleeding should have a group and hold
Creatinine kinase (CK)	With muscle death CK will rise
Microbiology	
Imaging	
Digital subtraction angiogram (DSA)	Can diagnose the occlusion and can potentially treat the issue, e.g. thrombolysis, angioplasty, clot retrieval
±CT angiogram / MR angiogram	If the patient is unable to have a DSA or if wanting to clarify diagnosis
Echocardiogram	May diagnose a left ventricular aneurysm or dilated thoracic aorta which potentially could be the source of embolus
Other	
Patch testing	Not required here, but if suspected allergic type reaction may consider
Excisional biopsy	Looking for malignancy

Diagnosis

Acute limb ischaemia

An acute presentation of limb pain in a vasculopathy with decreased ABI is very concerning for acute limb ischaemia and must be urgently reviewed by a vascular surgeon.

The gold standard investigation to confirm acute limb ischaemia is digital subtraction angiogram.

Discussion

Remember the 6 Ps of limb ischaemia: Pallor, Pain, Pulselessness, Paraesthesia, Perishingly cold, Paralysis.

Management

Medical

- Conservative management (not indicated here unless patient was not suitable for any surgical intervention / refused treatment)

- Nil by mouth
- IV fluids
- Heparin infusion
- Antiplatelet therapy
- Statin
- Pentoxifylline
- Analgesia

Surgical

- Revascularisation that may include endovascular with DSA, angioplasty ± stent and thrombolysis

- Surgical embolectomy or surgical bypass
- Following revascularisation if prolonged period of ischaemia or suspicious of compartment syndrome, should consider fasciotomy ± debridement of necrotic tissue; antibiotics should be given
- If irreversible ischaemia is encountered or treatment failure, amputation can be carried out

Other differential diagnoses

- Chronic limb ischaemia
- L5 or S1 radiculopathy secondary to foraminal stenosis or disc prolapse

Station 26 **Foot ulcer**

A 67-year-old woman presents to the GP with a long history of non-healing wounds on her feet.

Tasks

1 Take a history and examination
2 Perform a targeted examination

3 Describe appropriate investigations
4 Formulate a management plan

Differential diagnoses (VIITAMINC)

Vascular:
- Varicose veins
- Arterial ulcers
- Vasculitis

Infective:
- Mycobacterial ulcer
- Staphylococcal infection
- Syphilis

Inflammatory:
- Peripheral neuropathy leading to ulcers
- Pyoderma gangrenosum
- Insect bite

Trauma

Autoimmune

Metabolic:
- Diabetic neuropathy leading to ulcers

Iatrogenic

Neoplastic:
- Leiomyosarcoma
- Melanoma
- Squamous cell carcinoma
- Marjolin's ulcer

Congenital

Other:
- Pressure injuries

Before starting

Establish rapport:
- Introduce yourself
- Obtain consent to take a history and examine the patient
- Exposure: when physical examination is required, inform the patient that the area you will examine is exposed appropriately

Confirm patient details:
- Name   *Jenny Easterbrook*
- Age   *67 years*
- Occupation   *Clothes shop manager*

History

Pain history (SOCRATES)
- **S**ite: *right ankle is sore; mostly over the outer part*
- **O**nset: *progressively worsened over the past few months*
- **C**haracter: *ache*
- **R**adiation: *general heaviness and aching of legs*
- **A**ssociation: *associated with a wound which doesn't seem to heal*
- **T**ime: *worse with standing*
- **E**xacerbating / relieving factors: *elevating legs seems to help*
- **S**everity: *2/10*

Vascular history

- Calf pain: *yes, aching in the legs*
- Skin colour changes in the lower limbs: *yes, pale with areas of different colour*
- Varicose veins: *yes*
- Irritation of skin in the legs: *yes*
- Previous wounds to the lower limbs: *has had similar in the past, though not as bad; usually quite shallow with change in skin colour around the ulcer site*
- Redness, discharge, enlarging, warmth: *no*
- Swelling in the legs: *yes, at the end of the day*
- Pain in the legs: *yes, generalised ache, worse on standing*
- Any pain in calves / back of leg when walking: *pain improves when moving about*
- Coolness or warmth of legs: *legs are cool*
- Any shooting pain: *no*

Take a focused history

- *Well otherwise*
- Loss of weight: *no*
- Fevers, sweats or chills: *no*
- Recent insect bites: *no*
- Recent travel / sick contacts: *no*

Past medical history and family history

- *Hypertension and type 2 diabetes mellitus (T2DM)*
- *Mother had something similar 10 years ago*

Drug history and allergies

- *Metformin*
- *NKDA*

Social history

- Smoking history: *15 pack-years*
- Alcohol and drugs history: *3 glasses of wine per day, nil illicit drugs*
- *Works as hairdresser, prolonged periods of standing is part of job*
- *At home with husband*

Examination

General inspection (ABCD-V)

- **A**ppearance: *patient is comfortable*
- **B**ody habitus: *normal, BMI 23*
- **C**ognition: *patient is oriented*
- **D**evices / **D**rugs: *nil aids*
- **V**itals: *all within normal limits*

Lower limb examination

- Inspection:
  - *No atrophy of muscles*
  - *No hair on lower legs*
  - *Skin is not pale, but it has some thickening and discolouration*
  - *There are obvious varicose veins and previous scars from previous ulceration*
  - *Lower limbs look like there is some mild swelling*
  - *There is an ulcer above the medial malleolus on the right ankle; it looks irregular approximately 3–4cm in maximal dimensions, with a shallow appearance; granulation at the base is seen*
- Palpation:
  - *Skin is warm*
  - *Good capillary refill*
  - *Pulses from abdominal aorta to distal are strong*
  - *Nil calf tenderness*
- Auscultation:
  - *Nil bruits heard from abdominal aorta to popliteal*
- Buerger's, Trendelenburg and Perthes tests: *normal*
- Ankle brachial index: *normal*
- *Normal power 5/5 and sensation; proprioception intact*

Investigations

BBMI-O: Bedside, **B**loods, **M**icrobiology, **I**maging and **O**ther

Investigation	Rationale
Bedside	
▨ Ankle brachial index	▨ To rule out arterial disease
Bloods	
▨ FBC, U&Es and creatinine, CRP	▨ Generally venous ulcers can be diagnosed clinically; unless there are concerns of infection, blood tests are not required
▨ Blood glucose level and HbA1c	▨ Looking for T2DM and its potential complications of peripheral neuropathy
▨ ANA, ANCA, C3/4, ESR, RF, cryoglobulins, ENA, lupus anticoagulant, anti-cardiolipin Ab, prothrombin gene mutation, protein C/S, APC resistance, factor V Leiden, homocysteine, etc.	▨ Other tests can be considered if it is thought that vasculitis or thrombophilia are the underlying cause for the ulcers
Microbiology	
▨ Wound MCS	▨ If concerns of infection, one may do a wound MCS
Imaging	
▨ ±Duplex US	▨ Assess the arterial/venous systems; excludes deep vein thrombosis; can assess for venous reflux
▨ ±Angiogram, e.g. CTA/MRA	▨ If concerns of arterial occlusion
Other	
▨ Patch testing	▨ Not required here, but if suspected allergic type reaction may consider
▨ Excisional biopsy	▨ Looking for malignancy

Diagnosis

Venous insufficiency ulcer

Pain improving on walking, prolonged periods of standing and a known family history with a relatively benign examination is suggestive of venous insufficiency.

Management

Medical

- Wound care / dressings
- Barrier cream for venous stasis dermatitis
- Compression stockings
- Aspirin / pentoxifylline – analgesia
- Elevation (reduces oedema) at least 30 minutes several times per day
- Treatment of exacerbating factors e.g. deep vein thrombosis

Surgical

- Skin grafting may be helpful for those who do not improve after medical therapy

Other differential diagnoses

- Arterial ulcer
- Diabetic ulcer
- Pressure ulcer

Station 27 **Gait disturbance**

A 65-year-old man is brought by his wife to the emergency department with a history of several months of increasing difficulty walking and increasing forgetfulness.

Tasks

1 Take a history
2 Perform a targeted examination
3 Describe appropriate investigations
4 Formulate a management plan

Differential diagnoses

Neurological:
- Parkinson's disease
- Normal pressure hydrocephalus (NPH)
- Progressive supranuclear palsy
- Huntington's disease
- Stroke
- Central nervous system tumours
- Vascular dementia
- Cerebellar ataxia, e.g. from cerebellar stroke, alcohol abuse, etc.
- Cervical / thoracic myelopathy
- Vertebrobasilar insufficiency
- Multiple sclerosis

Sensory:
- Hearing impairment
- Vestibular neuritis
- Benign paroxysmal positional vertigo (BPPV)
- Peripheral neuropathy
- Visual impairment

Musculoskeletal:
- Myopathies / myositis
- Osteoarthritis
- Osteomyelitis
- Trauma
- Rheumatoid arthritis
- Dermatomyositis
- Gout
- Lumbar canal stenosis
- Spinal foraminal stenosis

Metabolic:
- Vitamin / mineral deficiencies, e.g. vitamin B_{12}
- Diabetic neuropathy

Cardiovascular:
- Congestive cardiac failure
- Peripheral artery disease
- Orthostatic hypotension

Before starting

Establish rapport:
- Introduce yourself
- Obtain consent to take a history and examine the patient
- Exposure: when physical examination is required, inform the patient that the area you will examine is exposed appropriately

Confirm patient details:
Name	*Ray Bond*
Age	*65 years*
Occupation	*Retired*

History

Neurological history

- Headache: *yes, constant headaches which have been worsening over the last few months*
- Nausea / vomiting: *no*
- Back or neck pain: *no*

- Shooting / radicular pain: *no*
- Lower limb pain: *no*
- Paraesthesia / numbness: *no*
- Change to urinary or bowel habits: *no*
- Weakness or sensory changes in the legs: *no*
- Changes to memory / cognition: *yes, worsening over last few months*
- Difficulty walking: *yes*
- Tremor: *no*

Other

- General health: *otherwise well*
- Shortness of breath: *no*
- Dizziness: *no*
- Arrhythmia: *no*
- Seizure-like activity: *no*
- Falls history: *yes, over the last few months; worsening as the walking difficulty progressed*
- Pre-syncopal and post-syncopal symptoms: *no*

Past medical history and family history

- Nil significant past medical history
- Father had osteoarthritis, mother had migraines

Drug history and allergies

- *Nil*
- *NKDA*

Social history

- Smoking history: *ex-smoker, 20 pack-years*

- Alcohol and drugs history: *social drinker, nil illicit drugs*
- *Retired; at home with wife*

Examination

General inspection (ABCD-V)

- **A**ppearance: *patient is comfortable*
- **B**ody habitus: *normal, BMI 23*
- **C**ognition: *patient is slightly confused; not oriented to place*
- **D**evices / **D**rugs: *patient has a 4-wheel frame*
- **V**itals: *all within normal limits*

Lower limb neurological examination

- Inspection of gait:
  - *Bradykinetic, wide-based gait, 'glue-footed'*
  - *Use of a 4-wheel frame*
- Romberg's negative
- Tone: *normal to slightly increased tone*
- Power: *5/5 throughout the lower limb*
- Reflexes: *increased ankle and knee reflexes; plantars downgoing*
- Coordination: *normal, no dysdiadochokinesis nor dysmetria*
- Sensation: *normal temperature, touch, prick, proprioception*

Investigations

BBMI-O: Bedside, **B**loods, **M**icrobiology, **I**maging and **O**ther

Investigation	Rationale
Bedside	
Bloods	
FBC	Looking for infection and anaemia
U&Es and creatinine	Looking for electrolyte imbalances and renal injury
Coagulation studies	Looking for coagulation profile in case patient is for an operation
±CRP	Looking for infection
±Syphilis testing – VDRL and RPR	Looking for tertiary syphilis involving the spinal cord

Investigation	Rationale
±Glucose level and HbA1c	Looking for diabetes mellitus and its potential complications of peripheral neuropathy
±B$_{12}$, vitamin E, copper deficiency	Low levels can be associated with subacute combined degeneration of spinal cord
Microbiology	
Imaging	
CT brain ± MRI brain	Looking for enlarged ventricles – Evans ratio >0.3 (maximum frontal horn ventricular width divided by the transverse inner diameter of the skull); MRI T2-weighted images can show high signal next to the ventricles showing transependymal cerebrospinal fluid transudation; dilation of the aqueduct
±MRI spine	Some upper motor neurone signs in this case; if suspecting spinal cord pathology causing symptoms, it would be reasonable to order an MRI spine
Other	
Timed up and go test in conjunction with lumbar puncture with high volume 40ml drained	Looking to quantitate patient's mobility pre and post lumbar puncture
Lumbar puncture	Looking for normal pressure and for high volume tap (high specificity); CSF MCS and biochemistry to exclude infectious causes
Lumbar drain	If a high-volume tap is inconclusive a lumbar drain has higher specificity and sensitivity to evaluate NPH; this is usually kept in for 2–3 days draining at approximately 10–15ml per hour (high specificity and sensitivity)

Diagnosis

Normal pressure hydrocephalus

An initial presentation of gait disturbance and cognition difficulties in a previously well patient fits more with the onset of NPH.

Management

Medical (not indicated here)

Surgical

- Ventricular shunting: this could be ventriculoperitoneal (most common) or ventriculoatrial or ventriculopleural shunt; other alternatives include lumboperitoneal shunting
- Those unsuitable for surgery may be offered repeated large-volume CSF taps and should be counselled on control of their vascular risk factors, e.g. smoking, blood pressure, cholesterol, etc., to prevent a vascular issue compounding their NPH

Other differential diagnoses

- Parkinson's disease
- Myelopathy
- Stroke
- Other dementias, e.g. Alzheimer's dementias

Station 28 **Goitre**

An 18-year-old woman presented to her GP with concerns of swelling in her neck.

Tasks

1 Take a history
2 Perform a targeted examination
3 Describe appropriate investigations
4 Formulate a management plan

Differential diagnoses

Metabolic:
- Thyroiditis
- Hashimoto's thyroiditis
- Graves' disease
- Solitary nodule
- Multinodular goitre

- Colloid nodule
- Sarcoidosis
- Iodine deficiency
- Thyroglossal cyst
- Adenoma
- Thyroid carcinoma

Before starting

Establish rapport:
- Introduce yourself
- Obtain consent to take a history and examine the patient
- Exposure: when physical examination is required, inform the patient that the area to be examined will be exposed appropriately

Confirm patient details:
- Name — *Stacey de la Hoyde*
- Age — *18 years*
- Occupation — *University student*

History

History of presenting complaint
- Onset: *4 months*
- Change in size / consistency: *increasing in size, no change in consistency*
- Changes to voice: *no*
- Difficulty breathing: *no*
- Cough: *no*
- Trouble swallowing: *no*
- Inappropriate hot / cold: *feels hot all the time, family states inappropriately dressed all the time*
- Change in weight: *lost 5kg over 4 months*
- Menstrual history: *has had irregular and scarce periods since symptoms started*
- Changes in bowel habits: *normal bowels, possibly increased in frequency*
- Fatigue: *no*
- Changes in appearance, hair or skin: *no*
- Palpitations: *yes*
- Uncontrollable shakes: *occasionally*
- Any recent cold / viral-type symptoms: *no*
- Painful or swollen neck: *no*
- Changes to vision: *no*

Past medical history and family history
- *Nil significant past medical history*
- *Mother has type 1 diabetes mellitus, maternal aunt has a 'thyroid problem'*

Drug history and allergies
- *Combined oral contraceptive pill*
- *NKDA*

Social history
- Smoking history: *non-smoker*
- Alcohol and drugs history: *social drinker, nil illicit drugs*

Examination

General inspection (ABCD-V)

▦ **A**ppearance: *patient is comfortable*
▦ **B**ody habitus: *normal BMI*
▦ **C**ognition: *patient is Glasgow Coma Scale (GCS) 15*
▦ **D**evices/**D**rugs: *nil*
▦ **V**itals: *BP 110/62mmHg, HR 108bpm regular, RR 16 per minute; oxygen saturation at 99% on room air; temperature 36.8°C*

Thyroid examination

▦ Inspection:
  ● Neck: *no scars, a large diffuse goitre, the goitre moves up and down with swallowing; voice is not hoarse*
  ● Face: *proptosis of the eyes and lid lag with eye movements*
  ● Limbs: *fingers show onycholysis, particularly of the 4th digits; lower limbs negative for pretibial myxoedema*
▦ Palpation of the neck: *the thyroid gland is smooth and diffusely enlarged; no nodules are palpable; the gland moves up and down on swallow; the thyroid is felt inferiorly*
▦ *Percussion of the sternum reveals no increased dullness; pressure on the thyroid does not cause stridor (Kocher's test negative); Pemberton's sign is negative*
▦ *No lymphadenopathy*
▦ *Reflexes throughout the upper and lower limbs are brisk*
▦ Auscultation of the thyroid: *you hear a bruit; heart sounds are dual with a mild regular tachycardia*

Investigations

BBMI-O: Bedside, **B**loods, **M**icrobiology, **I**maging and **O**ther

Investigation	Rationale
Bedside	
▦ ECG	▦ To ensure nil arrhythmias
Bloods	
▦ FBC	▦ Baseline as treatment, e.g. carbimazole, can cause haematological effects
▦ U&Es and creatinine	▦ Looking for renal injury
▦ ±Coagulation studies	▦ Looking for coagulation profile when the patient is for an operation
▦ Thyroid function tests T_3/T_4, TBG and TSH	▦ In Graves' T_3 and T_4 are elevated with low–normal TSH
▦ Thyroid antibodies (TSH receptor antibodies, anti-TPO, anti-thyroglobulin)	▦ TSH receptor is Ab-positive in Graves' disease
▦ ±CMP	▦ If the patient is for a surgery should get a baseline calcium phosphate level
▦ ±Beta-hCG	▦ In females of reproductive age, when planning to treat with radioactive iodine
▦ ±LFTs	▦ If undergoing treatment baseline LFTs are helpful as some medications can derange LFTs

Investigation	Rationale
Microbiology	
Imaging	
Ultrasound ± FNA	Can show large thyroid with increased vascularity, estimates thyroid volume as well for radioactive iodine treatment; if suspicious lesion seen can be biopsied
±CT orbits	If unclear cause of proptosis is noted
Tc-99m scan or I-123 thyroid scan	Homogeneous increased uptake; can see hot and cold areas; cold areas may be considered for biopsy
Chest and neck X-rays	May see retrosternal extension
Other	

Diagnosis

Graves' disease

A young patient with clinical signs of hyperthyroidism and particularly Graves' eye signs is highly suggestive of the disease.

Management

Multiple options are possible:

Medical

- Beta blockers to reduce heart rate / symptomatic thyrotoxicosis
- Antithyroid medications, i.e. carbimazole, with monitoring of TFTs and titration OR carbimazole higher dose with thyroxine when euthyroid
- Radioactive iodine and steroids

Surgical

- Total / near-total thyroidectomy

Other differential diagnoses

- De Quervain's thyroiditis
- Drug-induced thyroiditis
- Toxic nodular goitre

Station 29 **Groin mass**

A 40-year-old man is brought to the emergency department by his work colleagues with worsening groin pain, associated with nausea and vomiting.

Tasks

1 Take a history
2 Perform a targeted examination

3 Describe appropriate investigations
4 Formulate a management plan

Differential diagnoses (VIITAMINC)

Vascular:
- Ischaemic colitis
- Abdominal aortic aneurysm (AAA)

Infective:
- Gastroenteritis
- Infective colitis
- Appendicitis
- Diverticulitis
- UTI / pyelonephritis
- Spontaneous bacterial peritonitis
- Epiploic appendicitis
- Familial Mediterranean fever

Inflammatory:
- Testicular torsion
- Torsion of testicular appendage
- Renal colic
- Intussusception
- Inflammatory bowel disease
- Irritable bowel syndrome
- Pseudo-obstruction

Trauma

Autoimmune

Metabolic:
- Hyponatraemia / electrolyte abnormalities
- Diabetic ketoacidosis
- Acute intermittent porphyria

Iatrogenic

Neoplastic:
- Malignancy

Congenital

Other:
- Small bowel / large bowel obstruction
- Obstruction secondary to incarcerated / strangulated hernia (direct, indirect inguinal, femoral, incisional, etc.)

Before starting

Establish rapport:
- Introduce yourself
- Obtain consent to take a history and examine the patient
- Expose the patient; when physical examination is required inform the patient that the area you will examine is exposed appropriately

Confirm patient details:
- Name   *Barry White*
- Age   *40 years*
- Occupation   *Construction worker*

History

Pain history (SOCRATES)

- **S**ite: *groin is very painful*
- **O**nset: *started this morning while at work carrying timber*

Character: *constant severe ache in the right groin*

Radiation: *some lower abdominal pain too*

Association: *had a lump here that usually comes and goes, but now it is quite prominent and not going away*

Time: *never had it before; just occurred today*

Exacerbating/relieving factors: *hasn't tried anything yet; just came to emergency department*

Severity: *9/10*

History of presenting complaint

Bowels last opened: *7am, normal formed movement*

Last flatus: *2 hours ago*

Nausea or vomiting: *no*

Fever/chills: *no*

Previous abdominal surgery: *no*

How long have you had a lump in your groin: *8 months*

Where is the lump: *right groin*

Time course of lump: *intermittent lump, currently constantly out*

What size is it normally: *1cm × 1cm*

What size is it now: *5cm × 4cm*

Weight training/heavy lifting: *yes, for work*

Last ate: *6:30am*

Urinary symptoms: *no*

Discharge from penis: *no*

Sexual history: *married 10 years, single sexual partner*

Past medical history and family history

Nil significant past medical history

Father has type 2 diabetes mellitus

Drug history and allergies

Nil

NKDA

Social history

Smoking history: *10 pack-years*

Alcohol and drugs history: *3 beers per day, occasional marijuana use*

At home with wife

Examination

General inspection (ABCD-V)

Appearance: *patient is uncomfortable*

Body habitus: *overweight, BMI 26*

Cognition: *patient is oriented*

Devices/**D**rugs: *nil*

Vitals: *BP 130/80mmHg, HR 102bpm, RR 19 per minute; oxygen saturation at 100% on room air; temperature 37.8°C*

Abdominal examination

Inspection: *nil previous scars; distended abdomen; erythematous tennis-ball-sized lump on the right groin*

Palpation: *abdomen distended but soft; right groin lump over inguinal region tender +++; unable to reduce the lump post analgesia*

Percussion: *resonant percussion*

Auscultation: *bowel sounds unable to hear*

Investigations

BBMI-O: Bedside, **B**loods, **M**icrobiology, **I**maging and **O**ther

Investigation	Rationale
Bedside	
Bloods	
FBC	Looking for inflammation, platelets
U&Es and creatinine	Looking for electrolyte imbalances and renal injury
Coagulation studies	Looking for coagulation profile in case patient is for an operation
±CRP	Looking for inflammation
ABG	Looking for lactate which can be raised in setting of bowel ischaemia

Investigation	Rationale
▨ Group and hold	▨ If patient is likely for operation
Microbiology	
Imaging	
▨ CT abdomen and pelvis	▨ If unsure or clinical findings of incarcerated / strangulated hernia is equivocal, may consider a CT abdomen and pelvis; may be more helpful in patients with high BMI; may show radiological features of small bowel obstruction, dilated bowel proximal to hernia site; may see bowel / omentum contents in hernia sac with free fluid, fat stranding, thickened bowel
▨ Abdominal X-ray	▨ May see abdominal X-ray features of bowel obstruction
Other	

Diagnosis

Strangulated inguinal hernia with small bowel obstruction

An irreducible hernia that is painful, associated with vomiting, is highly suspicious for small bowel obstruction.

Management

Medical

▨ Analgesia
▨ IV fluids
▨ Fasting status (patient will require surgery for definitive management)

Surgical

▨ Inguinal hernia repair ± mesh (should not put in if bowel ischaemia is present) ± laparotomy and bowel resection

▨ Patient should also be informed they may have a potential stoma if bowel resection is needed and anastomosis is not possible

Other differential diagnoses

▨ Femoral hernia ± strangulated
▨ Hydrocele
▨ Testicular torsion
▨ Epididymo-orchitis

Station 30 **Gynaecomastia**

An 18-year-old man presented to his GP concerned about increasing breast size with associated pain over the past 2–3 months.

Tasks

1 Take a history
2 Perform a targeted examination

3 Describe appropriate investigations
4 Formulate a management plan

Differential diagnoses (VIITAMINC)

Vascular

Infective

Inflammatory:
- Liver cirrhosis
- Renal disease

Trauma

Autoimmune

Metabolic:
- Pituitary adenoma – prolactinoma
- Adrenal carcinoma
- Testicular tumour:
  - Leydig or Sertoli cell
  - Germ cell tumours

- Hypogonadism, e.g. Klinefelter's syndrome, trauma, hereditary defects of androgen synthesis, orchitis
- Physiological
- Puberty
- Hyperthyroidism

Iatrogenic

Neoplastic:
- Hepatocellular carcinoma

Congenital

Other:
- Drug-related, i.e. cimetidine, spironolactone, marijuana, anabolic steroids, oestrogen, thiazide diuretics
- Idiopathic

Before starting

Establish rapport:
- Introduce yourself
- Obtain consent from the patient: "I'll be asking you questions to find out the reasons behind your concerns today"
- Expose the patient: when physical examination is required, inform the patient that the area you will examine is exposed appropriately

Confirm patient details:
- Name   *Ben Dawes*
- Age   *18 years*
- Occupation   *University student*

History

Pain history (SOCRATES)
- **S**ite: *general breast tissue bilaterally*
- **O**nset: *2–3 months ago*
- **C**haracter: *dull ache, more specific tenderness on palpation over nipples*
- **R**adiation: *no*
- **A**ssociated symptoms: *no*
- **T**ime/duration: *constant*
- **E**xacerbating/relieving factors: *no*
- **S**everity: *2–3/10 constant, 4–5/10 on palpation over nipple*

History of presenting complaint

- Change in the nipple: *no*
- Discharge from nipple: *no*
- Alcohol / drug history: *no medications, alcohol intake 3–4 standard units per week; patient is a current marijuana user – 2 joints per day*
- Lumps in the testes / recent trauma to testes: *no*
- Change to libido / erection maintenance: *normal, no issues*
- Loss of weight: *no*
- Changes to vision: *no*

Past medical history

- Nil significant past medical history
- Nil family history

Drug history and allergies

- Nil
- NKDA

Social history

- Smoking: *2 pack-years*
- Alcohol and drugs history: *as above*
- Living on campus

Examination

General inspection (ABCD-V)

- **A**ppearance: *patient is comfortable*

- **B**ody habitus: *normal, BMI 23*
- **C**ognition: *patient is Glasgow Coma Scale (GCS) 15*
- **D**evices / **D**rugs: *nil*
- **V**itals: *all within normal limits*

Breast examination

Ask the patient to lie down, explain clearly that the breasts will need to be examined. Ask for a chaperone to be present (if available).

- Inspection (look for enlarged breast size, any asymmetry, nipple retraction or discharge): *enlarged breasts noted, otherwise no abnormalities*
- Palpation:
  - Ensure all four quadrants of the breast are palpated with the pulps of your fingers; looking for any lumps or area of tenderness
  - *On palpation of the breast areolar complex, a firm tissue is felt; placing a thumb and finger together a 2cm firmness symmetrical bilaterally which is mildly tender*

Testicular examination

Unremarkable

Investigations

BBMI-O: Bedside, **B**loods, **M**icrobiology, **I**maging and **O**ther

Investigation	Rationale
Bedside	
Bloods	
FBC	Looking for anaemia
U&Es and creatinine	Looking for renal injury
Coagulation studies	Looking for coagulation profile if / when patient is for an operation
Thyroid function tests	If suspicious of hyperthyroidism
LFTs	If suspicious of chronic liver disease
AFP	If suspicious of hepatocellular carcinoma

Investigation	Rationale
▨ Beta-hCG, DHEA, testosterone, LH, FSH	▨ If suspicious of adrenal / testicular pathology
▨ PRL	▨ If suspicious of prolactinoma
Microbiology	
Imaging	
▨ Mammogram or US of the breast ± FNA	▨ If clinical history and examination is suspicious for breast cancer
▨ Testicular US	▨ If clinical examination and examination is suspicious for testicular cancer and oestradiol is raised
Other	

Diagnosis

Drug-induced (marijuana) gynaecomastia

Gynaecomastia in a patient with nil other symptoms, a normal BMI and a benign examination indicates that the likely cause is his drug use.

Management

Medical

- ▨ In this patient, it would be appropriate to advise against marijuana use and provide reassurance
- ▨ If resolution did not occur, it may be worth a trial of tamoxifen or clomiphene

Surgical

- ▨ Can be considered in cases where a considerable psychological impact is experienced by the patient

- ▨ Multiple techniques; however, most commonly used is the subcutaneous mastectomy

Other differential diagnoses

- ▨ Pseudogynaecomastia (i.e. obesity-induced)
- ▨ Breast cancer (uncommon in males)
- ▨ Physiological gynaecomastia

Station 31 **Haematemesis**

A 62-year-old woman presents to the emergency department after an acute episode of nausea, followed by vomiting one cup of blood.

Tasks

1 Take a history
2 Perform a targeted examination
3 Describe appropriate investigations
4 Formulate a management plan

Differential diagnoses (VIITAMINC)

Vascular:
- Oesophageal varices
- Dieulafoy's lesion
- Angiodysplasia
- Watermelon stomach – antral vascular ectasia
- Coagulopathy

Infective

Inflammatory:
- Peptic ulcer disease – chronic or acute
- Oesophagitis

Trauma:
- Mallory–Weiss tear

Autoimmune

Metabolic

Iatrogenic

Neoplastic:
- Malignancy

Congenital:
- Arteriovenous malformations

Other:
- Boerhaave syndrome

Before starting

In the setting of acute blood loss with unknown status of ongoing bleed, ensure the patient is adequately resuscitated and stable (**ABCDE**):
- **A**irway: *patient is conscious and alert; conversing in normal sentences; maintaining own airway*
- **B**reathing: *RR 14 per minute; oxygen saturation at 97% on room air; chest clear on auscultation, good air entry bilaterally with equal chest expansion*
- **C**irculation: *patient appears a little pale; HR 100bpm with BP 110/70mmHg; ECG shows sinus rhythm*
- **D**isability: *Glasgow Coma Scale (GCS) 15; pupils are equal and reactive to light*
- **E**xposure: *warm peripheries; no signs of peritonitis or acute abdomen (to suggest perforation) on examination*

Ensure patient is not reporting symptoms suggesting severe ongoing bleed:
- Dizziness
- Shortness of breath
- Chest pain, palpitations
- Cold and clammy peripheries

Establish rapport:
- Introduce yourself
- Consent the patient: "I'll be asking you some questions regarding your symptoms and some details about your past medical history. Later I will also be examining your abdomen.

Because you've experienced bleeding in your gastrointestinal tract, I will also need to perform a rectal check with your permission"; (per rectal exam is theoretical in an OSCE station)

- Expose the patient: when physical examination is required, it will require shirt / top to be taken off

Confirm patient details:
- Name   *Denise Makumbi*
- Age   *62 years*
- Occupation   *Hair stylist*

History

History of presenting complaint

Patient was using the computer at rest this evening. Had sudden wave of nausea and vomited in bathroom. Noted content of vomit was entirely blood.

- Onset: *sudden, acute*
- Description of blood: *dark red, mostly coffee ground in appearance*
- Associated symptoms: *nausea, dizziness, now resolved; mild abdominal discomfort now resolved; did not lose consciousness*
- Description of stools: *denies melaena or per rectal bleed*
- Previous episodes: *none*
- Constitutional symptoms: *none*

Past medical history and family history

- *Previous gastritis and treatment for* Helicobacter pylori
- *Denies previous abdominal surgeries*
- *Nil family history*

Drug history and allergies

- *Aspirin – GP started this; meloxicam – recently started taking for knee pain*
- *NKDA*

Social history

- Smoking history: *15 pack-years*
- Alcohol and drugs history: *non-drinker, nil illicit drugs*

Examination

General inspection (ABCD-V)

- **A**ppearance: *patient looks well*
- **B**ody habitus: *overweight, BMI 28*
- **C**ognition: *patient is conscious and oriented*
- **D**evices / **D**rugs: *hypertension tablets on table and the patient is wearing nasal prongs with 2 L oxygen flow*
- **V**itals: *BP 140/90mmHg, HR 95bpm and regular; other vital signs are within normal range*

Abdominal examination

- Inspection:
  - Skin: *no jaundice or spider naevi (liver disease); no ecchymoses (coagulopathy) or petechiae (alcoholism)*
  - Hands: *no palmar erythema (liver disease); no telangiectasia (hereditary haemorrhagic telangiectasia); no palmar pallor (anaemia)*
  - Abdomen: *no distension; no caput medusae (liver disease); no scars or signs of previous abdominal surgery*
- Palpation: superficial and deep palpation:
  - *Mild epigastric tenderness*
  - *Soft abdomen; no guarding or signs of peritonism*
  - *No masses palpable; no organomegaly*
- Percussion: *resonant*
- Auscultation: *bowel sounds present*

Digital rectal examination

- External: *no abnormalities*
- Internal: *no masses palpable; light brown faeces on glove; no blood*

Investigations

BBMI-O: Bedside, **B**loods, **M**icrobiology, **I**maging and **O**ther

Investigation	Rationale
Bedside	
Bloods	
FBC	Assess haemoglobin
U&Es and creatinine	Assess renal function
Coagulation profile	Screening for coagulopathy
LFTs	Screening for liver disease
Group and hold	Pre-empting need for blood transfusion
Microbiology	
Imaging	
CXR	Screening for perforated ulcer
CT angiography	To assess active source of bleed (if unclear on history)
Other	
Endoscopy ± biopsy	To identify source of bleeding
Colonoscopy ± biopsy	Looking for areas of thickened bowel wall, inflamed bowel wall; positive biopsies would be indicative of malignancy

Diagnosis

Peptic ulcer disease

A patient with history of peptic ulcer disease and recent NSAID use is highly suspicious for peptic ulcer disease.

The gold standard investigation to confirm peptic ulcer disease is endoscopy ± biopsy.

Management

Resuscitation

- IV fluid replacement
- Blood transfusion: if haemoglobin low, haemodynamically unstable despite fluid resuscitation, or severe active bleed
- Platelet transfusion: if thrombocytopenic
- Fresh frozen plasma: if non-cirrhotic elevated INR

Medication

- Proton pump inhibitor infusion for acid suppression
- Tranexamic acid for antifibrinolytic effects

Endoscopy

- Gastroscopy: diagnostic and therapeutic to identify and control source of bleeding: cautery, adrenaline or saline injection, mechanical clips, haemostatic spray

Operative

- If failed endoscopic and medical therapy; ongoing bleed with haemodynamic instability and anaemia
- Vagotomy
  - Removes branches of the vagus nerve to reduce gastric acid secretion

- Gastrectomy + reconstruction of the stomach
  - Antrectomy: removes the antrum (hormone stimulation)
  - Subtotal gastrectomy: eliminates number of parietal cells (acid-secretion)

Other differential diagnoses

- Oesophageal varices
- Mallory–Weiss tear

Station 32 **Haematuria**

A 67-year-old man presents to his GP complaining about difficulty in urinating and a sense of incomplete voiding, associated with blood in his urine.

Tasks

1 Take a history
2 Perform a targeted examination

3 Describe appropriate investigations
4 Formulate a management plan

Differential diagnoses (VIITAMINC)

Vascular:
- Coagulopathy

Infective:
- Urinary tract infection
- Pyelonephritis

Inflammatory:
- Renal calculi
- Glomerulonephritis

Trauma:
- Trauma to urinary tract

Autoimmune:
- Systemic lupus erythematosus

Metabolic

Iatrogenic:
- Medication-induced

Neoplastic:
- Benign prostatic hyperplasia
- Prostate cancer
- Bladder cancer
- Metastatic cancer

Congenital:
- Sickle cell anaemia

Other:
- Menstruation

Before starting

Establish rapport:
- Introduce yourself
- Consent the patient: "I'll be asking you some questions regarding your symptoms, and then I will need to examine your abdomen and groin area. I will also need to check your prostate via a rectal examination, with your permission"
- Expose the patient: when physical examination is required, it will require shirt / vest to be taken off

Confirm patient details:
- Name   *Bob Sheers*
- Age   *67 years*
- Occupation   *Postman*

History

History of presenting complaint

- *Patient reports 6-month history of increasing difficulty voiding; notices red discoloured urine in the bowl*
- Onset: *over 6 months*
- Description of blood: *bright red blood in urine*
- Associated symptoms:
  - *Reports frequency, nocturia, hesitancy, decreased stream, incomplete voiding*
  - *Denies polyuria, dysuria, incontinence, froth in urine, renal colic, abdominal pain, fever*
- Description of stools: *denies melaena or per rectal bleed*

▓ Trauma: *none; no recent surgery*
▓ Constitutional symptoms:
  ● *Unintentional weight loss*
  ● *Lethargy*
  ● *No night sweats*

Past medical history and family history

▓ *Hypertension, hypercholesterolaemia*
▓ *Father had benign prostatic hypertrophy*
▓ Prostate check / prostate-specific antigen (PSA): *never examined / tested*

Drug history and allergies

▓ *Amlodipine, rosuvastatin*
▓ *NKDA*

Social history

▓ Smoking history: *20 pack-years*
▓ Alcohol and drugs history: *4–5 standard units per week, nil illicit drugs*

Examination

General inspection (ABCD-V)

▓ **A**ppearance: *patient looks comfortable*
▓ **B**ody habitus: *normal, BMI 21*

▓ **C**ognition: *patient is conscious and oriented*
▓ **D**evices / **D**rugs: *nil*
▓ **V**itals: *BP 125/84mmHg, HR 70bpm and regular; afebrile*

Palpate

▓ Abdomen:
  ● *Soft, non-tender; no renal angle or suprapubic tenderness; no masses or organomegaly*
  ● Balloting: *nil palpable kidneys*
  ● Auscultation: *nil renal bruits*
▓ Genital exam:
  ● *Scrotum and penis do not look abnormal; no blood at meatus*
  ● *Testes smooth, firm, non-tender, equal in size*
  ● *No varicocele*
▓ PR exam:
  ● Prostate: *asymmetric with a unilateral hard nodule; no sulcus apparent; non-tender*
  ● *Brown faeces on glove, no blood*

Investigations

BBMI-O: Bedside, **B**loods, **M**icrobiology, **I**maging and **O**ther

Investigation	Rationale
Bedside	
Bloods	
▓ FBC	▓ Assess haemoglobin in the setting of haematuria
▓ U&Es and creatinine	▓ Assess renal function
▓ PSA	▓ Screening for disseminated prostate cancer
▓ Coagulation profile	▓ Screening for coagulopathy
▓ LFTs	▓ Screening for hepatitis (work-up for androgren deprivation therapy)
▓ Testosterone	▓ Work-up for androgren deprivation therapy
▓ Group and hold	▓ Pre-empting need for blood transfusion

Investigation	Rationale
Microbiology	
Imaging	
▦ CT abdomen and pelvis	▦ For staging; to asses pelvic lymph nodes
▦ MRI pelvis	▦ For staging; to assess for metastasis
▦ Bone scan	▦ Assessing for bone metastasis
Other	

Diagnosis

Prostate cancer

This patient is in the correct age group, has cancer risk factors and has a hard nodule felt over the prostate on examination. Until proven otherwise, prostate cancer is the primary differential.

The gold standard investigation to confirm prostate cancer is a biopsy.

Management

▦ Transrectal US-guided biopsy of prostate:
  - 10–12 cores are sampled (half from each side)
  - Gleason score is generated from biopsy result
▦ TNM staging:
  - Post biopsy, in conjunction with Gleason score
  - As per the imaging investigations above

Resultant treatment based on:

Patient's risk group, projected survival and patient preference
▦ Localised prostate cancer:
  - Radiotherapy

- Radical prostatectomy:
  ▸ Retropubic or perineal approach
  ▸ Include pelvic lymph node dissection
  ▸ The prostate, capsule, seminal vesicles, ampulla and vas deferens are removed
▦ Disseminated disease:
  - Androgen deprivation therapy (ADT):
    ▸ Gonadotrophin-releasing hormone agonist (medical castration)
  - Bilateral orchiectomy (surgical castration)
  - Immunotherapy, chemotherapy: for ADT-resistant disease

Other differential diagnoses

▦ Benign prostatic hyperplasia (BPH)
▦ Renal calculi

Station 33 **Haemoptysis**

An 85-year-old woman presents to the emergency department as she has been unwell for a few days with a cough, though today she has also noticed some blood.

Tasks

1 Take a history
2 Perform a targeted examination
3 Describe appropriate investigations
4 Formulate a management plan

Differential diagnoses (VIITAMINC)

Vascular:
- Pulmonary embolism
- Pulmonary arteriovenous malformation
- Mitral stenosis
- Bronchial telangiectasia
- Left ventricular failure

Infective:
- Bronchiectasis
- Acute / chronic bronchitis
- Pneumonia
- Fungal infection
- Lung abscess
- Tuberculosis

Inflammatory

Traumatic

Autoimmune:
- Systemic lupus erythematosus
- Goodpasture's syndrome

- Granulomatosis with polyangiitis
- Diffuse alveolar haemorrhage

Metabolic

Iatrogenic

Neoplastic:
- Primary lung cancer
- Lung metastases
- Bronchial adenoma

Coagulopathy:
- Anticoagulant or antiplatelet use
- Platelet dysfunction
- Disseminated intravascular coagulation (DIC)
- Thrombocytopenia

Other:
- Lung contusion / penetrating injury
- Toxic inhalation
- Aspiration of foreign body

Before starting

Establish rapport:
- Introduce yourself
- Consent the patient: "Would you be happy for me to ask you some questions about why you're here, and then perform a physical examination after?"
- Expose the patient when physical examination is required – this will require shirt / top to be taken off

Confirm patient details:

Name	*Shelly Temple*
Age	*85 years*
Occupation	*Retired, previously a nurse*

History

History of presenting complaint (SOCRATES)

- **S**ite: *cough and associated pain across the chest*
- **O**nset: *over the past 2 days*

Character: *sharp pain*

Radiation: *none*

Associated symptoms: *haemoptysis, fevers, rigors and chills since yesterday, confusion (can't seem to remember the day or time which is not baseline)*

Time: *consistent throughout the day*

Exacerbating / relieving: *pain worse when breathing in and coughing, nil relieving factors*

Severity: *limiting day-to-day activities*

Take a focused history

- Respiratory:
  - Breathing: *difficult, hard to take a full breath*
  - Cough: *yes, started 3 days ago, has been getting worse*
  - Coughing up phlegm / blood: *yes – changed from baseline amount, initially white but now increased amounts of mucus that is a yellow / green colour; noticed this morning it had blood streaks in it, the amount of blood has been getting worse; approximately 5ml total*
  - Wheeze: *moderate amount, more than baseline*
  - Postnasal drip: *no*
  - Hoarse voice: *no*
- Cardiovascular:
  - Lower limb oedema: *no*
  - Orthopnoea / paroxysmal nocturnal dyspnoea: *no*
  - Decreased exercise tolerance: *yes*
  - Syncope / light-headedness: *no*
  - Calf pain: *no*
- Systemic (**SWIM**):
  - **S**kin: *nil easy bruising nor tendency to bleed*
  - **W**eight: *no recent unexplained loss of weight or night sweats*
  - **I**nfective:
    - Fevers / sweats / rigors: *yes*
    - Sick contacts: *yes, husband had similar symptoms last week, however his symptoms have improved*
    - Coryzal symptoms or recent viral illness: *not prior to symptom onset*
    - Recent overseas travel: *no*
  - **M**usculoskeletal:
    - Joint pain: *no*
    - History of trauma: *no*

Past medical history and family history

- *Recurrent chest infections, chronic obstructive pulmonary disease (COPD), diabetes, hypertension*
- *Mother had COPD and had a heart attack at age 90 years, father had type 2 diabetes mellitus and hypertension*
- *Family history of malignancy: no*

Drug history and allergies

- *Salbutamol inhaler PRN, Seretide, metformin, perindopril*
- *NKDA*

Social history

- Smoking history: *yes, 40 pack-years*
- Alcohol and drugs history: *none*
- *Lives at home with her husband*
- *Requires support from family and once weekly community help*
- *Requires a 4-wheel frame*
- *Independent with activities of daily living usually, though currently struggling to keep up*

Examination

General inspection (ABCD-V)

- **A**ppearance: *patient looks uncomfortable and diaphoretic*
- **B**ody habitus: *normal, BMI 22*
- **C**ognition: *patient is conscious and oriented*
- **D**evices / **D**rugs: *nil*
- **V**itals: *BP 130/70mmHg, HR 70bpm and regular, RR 22 per minute; oxygen saturation 96% on room air; febrile at 38.8°C*

Respiratory

- Inspection:
  - *Patient looks to be dyspnoeic, though no tripoding / accessory muscle use and diaphoretic*
  - *Able to speak in short sentences*
  - *Cough present – note the mucus cup next to the bed with greenish sputum and a tinge of blood through it*
  - *No presence of cyanosis, scars or chest wall abnormalities*
  - *No clubbing, peripheral cyanosis or asterixis*

Palpation:
- Trachea: *midline, no tug present*
- Cervical and supraclavicular lymph nodes: *non-palpable*
- Chest expansion: *symmetrical; Hoover's sign negative*
- Chest wall *non-tender*

Percussion:
- *Resonance in the apices bilaterally*
- *Dullness to percuss over the left lower zone, in comparison to right*

Auscultation:
- *Coarse crackles in the left lower zone*

- *Moderate expiratory wheeze globally*
- *Vocal resonance: increased in left lower zone*

Cardiovascular:

Inspection: *no surgical scars, deformities or visible pulsations; apex beat not visualised*

Palpation: *apex beat not displaced, mid-clavicular 5th intercostal; no thrills or heaves are felt*

Percussion: *no effusions notable; no dullness to percussion at posterior chest*

Auscultation: *dual heart sounds with no murmurs*

Investigations

BBMI-O: Bedside, **B**loods, **M**icrobiology, **I**maging and **O**ther

Investigation	Rationale
Bedside	
Bloods	
FBC	Looking for infection and anaemia
CRP	Looking for infection / inflammation
U&Es and creatinine	Looking for electrolyte imbalances and renal injury
ABG	Looking at haemodynamic status in severe haemoptysis
Tumour markers (CEA / CA-125)	Looking for raised serum levels to suggest the development of lung cancer
Blood cultures	Looking for pathogen causing sepsis
Pathogen specific antigens: IgM, Legionella urinary antigen assay, pneumococcal urinary antigen assay	Looking for pathogens *Mycoplasma pneumoniae*, *Legionella* and *Streptococcus pneumoniae*
Microbiology	
Sputum MCS	Looking for infective organisms as a cause
NAAT (nucleic acid amplification testing) nose / throat swab	Looking for viral pathogens (i.e. influenza) and some bacterial pathogens (i.e. *Chlamydophila pneumoniae*)
Imaging	
CXR (PA and lateral views)	Looking for evidence of consolidation in infection, shadowing of lesions in cancer or abscesses
CT chest	Looking for evidence of lung lesions or abscesses

Investigation	Rationale
▨ PET scan	▨ Utilised in staging of cancer
▨ CT angiography	▨ Looking to determine the bleeding site
Other	
▨ Bronchoscopy	▨ Looking for the causative bleeding site and source; therapeutic intervention to stop the bleeding
▨ ECHO	▨ Looking at baseline cardiac function if surgery is required and for cardiac causes

Diagnosis

Community-acquired pneumonia

Examination findings of coarse crackles on the left compared with the right, in conjunction with decreased percussion note and increased vocal resonance is suggestive of consolidation in that lung. This, combined with fever and a history of COPD and recurrent chest infections, puts this patient at high risk of pneumonia.

The gold standard investigation to confirm pneumonia is a sputum microscopy, culture and sensitivity (MCS) in conjunction with CXR.

Discussion

Pneumonia is inflammation of the lungs with consolidation or interstitial infiltrates.

Community-acquired pneumonia (CAP): pneumonia that develops from infection outside a hospital or healthcare facility. The most common cause is *Streptococcus pneumoniae*, with *Mycoplasma pneumoniae* being a major cause of atypical bacterial pneumonia.

Hospital-acquired pneumonia (HAP): pneumonia arising at least 48 hours after admission to a hospital / health facility, where the disease was not present at the time of admission.

Ventilator-associated pneumonia (VAP) is defined as pneumonia occurring more than 48 hours post endotracheal intubation.

Management

Haemoptysis

▨ Emergency response protocol: DRSABCD

▨ Maintain patent airway:
- Positioning
- Chin lift / jaw thrust
- Airway adjuncts (i.e. Guedel)
- Endotracheal tube

▨ Resuscitation:
- Bleeding lung side down; if both sides bleeding place head down
- Isolate lung (i.e. railroad endotracheal tube into the non-bleeding lung with endoscope or place double lumen endotracheal tube)

▨ Fluid resuscitation

▨ Blood product replacement (if severe haemorrhage or symptomatic)

▨ Treat bleeding source:
- Correct coagulopathy (if indicated)
- Bronchial artery embolisation
- Bronchoscopic laser photocoagulation
- Iced normal saline lavage (of involved lung segments)
- Topical adrenaline
- IV vasopressin

- Surgical resection / occlusion of offending vessel

Pneumonia (CAP)

- Lifestyle:
  - Stop smoking / excessive alcohol consumption (aspiration risk)
  - Vaccinations annually (i.e. influenza and pneumococcus)
  - Adequate nutrition
- Medical:
  - Analgesia as required
  - Oxygen therapy if indicated
  - Cough suppressant (i.e. codeine if uncontrollable coughing)
  - Antipyretics (i.e. paracetamol if fever)
  - Antibiotics: route, type and duration dependent on severity of disease (see below)
- Surgical:
  - Incision and drainage of abscess (if indicated)

Antibiotic therapy

Inpatient:
- Moderate:
  - Benzylpenicillin 1.2g IV QDS (until significant improvement) then change to amoxicillin 1g orally TDS for 7 days total course
    ▸ Ceftriaxone or cefotaxime IV then cefuroxime orally if hypersensitive to penicillins
  - PLUS: oral doxycycline 100mg BD, 7 days

- Severe:
  - Ceftriaxone 1g IV daily or cefotaxime 1g IV TDS
  - PLUS: azithromycin 500mg IV daily
  - Once clinically stable downgrade to oral therapy as per moderate

CURB 65

Scoring system that estimates the severity of pneumonia, assisting in determining if the patient undertakes an inpatient or outpatient treatment pathway:
- **C**onfusion
- **U**rea (>7mmol/L)
- **R**espiratory rate >30 per minute
- **B**lood pressure: systolic <90mmHg or diastolic <60mmHg
- **65:** age greater than 65 years

Score	Treatment
0–1	Outpatient care
2	Inpatient versus period of observation
3–5	Inpatient admission, with consideration of ICU admission if score 4–5

Other differential diagnoses

- Acute / chronic bronchitis
- Primary lung cancer

Station 34 **Hand pain**

A 60-year-old female presents to the GP with a 1-month history of unilateral wrist pain.

Tasks

1 Take a history
2 Perform physical examination

3 Describe appropriate investigations
4 Formulate a management plan

Differential diagnoses (VIITAMINC)

Vascular

Infective

Inflammatory:
- Rheumatoid arthritis
- Gout / pseudogout
- Psoriatic arthritis
- Reactive arthritis
- Osteoarthritis
- Amyloidosis
- Neuropathy
- Tendinopathy
- Tenosynovitis

Trauma:
- Ligament tears
- Distal radius / ulna fractures

- Carpal fractures
- Non-union of old injury

Autoimmune:
- Enteropathic arthropathy

Metabolic

Iatrogenic

Neoplastic

Congenital

Other:
- Avascular necrosis of carpal bones

Before starting

Establish rapport:
- Introduce yourself
- Consent the patient: "I'll be asking you some questions regarding your hand pain, then I'll examine your hand and ask you to do a few movements; would that be OK?"
- Expose the patient: when physical examination is required; as hands and wrists are usually already exposed, take the time to ensure you and your patient are positioned comfortably and each hand is easily accessible for examination and manipulations

Confirm patient details:
Name	*Sally Harris*
Age	*60 years*
Occupation	*Homemaker*

History

Pain history (SOCRATES)

- **S**ite: *right wrist palmar aspect*
- **O**nset: *insidious*
- **C**haracter: *dull, aching*
- **R**adiation: *short radiation proximally into forearm*

Associated symptoms: *paraesthesia of the first 3.5 digits (median nerve entrapment in carpal tunnel)*

Time / duration: *transient; can occur during the night*

Exacerbating / relieving factors: *exacerbated by actions involving repetitive flexion and extension of the wrist; can be relieved by shaking the hand*

Severity: *moderately intense; very uncomfortable; impedes use of involved hands*

Musculoskeletal and rheumatological history

- Any preceding trauma to the region: *no*
- Other joint involvement: *no*
- Constitutional symptoms: *no*
- Neurological symptoms: *paraesthesia in lateral 3.5 fingers*
- Any skin changes: *no*

Past medical history and family history

- *Type 2 diabetes mellitus*
- *Nil family history*

Drug history and allergies

- *Metformin*
- *Allergic to penicillins – anaphylaxis*

Social history

- Smoking history: *non-smoker*
- Alcohol and drugs history: *social drinker, nil illicit drugs*

Examination

General inspection (ABCD-V)

- **A**ppearance: *patient is in pain and moderately dyspnoeic*
- **B**ody habitus: *overweight, BMI 26*
- **C**ognition: *patient is conscious and oriented*
- **D**evices / **D**rugs: *no*
- **V**itals: *BP 120/80mmHg, HR 65bpm and regular; other vital signs are within normal range*

Rheumatological examination

- Inspection:
  - Skin: *normal colour, no previous scars / wounds*
  - Deformity: *no change to bony angulation and alignment, no muscle contractures*
  - Swelling: *no gross swelling*
  - Muscle atrophy: *mild atrophy of the right thenar prominence may be present*
  - Associated joints: *normal appearance of forearm and elbow*
- Palpation:
  - Masses: *none*
  - Temperature: *normal*
  - Tenderness: *mild discomfort over dorsum of wrist; no bony tenderness*
    - Anatomical snuffbox: *no scaphoid tenderness*
  - Effusion: *none*
  - Crepitus: *none*
  - Muscle bulk: *mild thenar atrophy*
  - Sensation: *intact*
  - Vascular / pulse: *radial and ulnar pulses present; capillary refill under 3 seconds*
- Movement:
  - Active:
    - Finger flexion, extension, abduction, adduction: *full proximal interphalangeal (PIP), distal interphalangeal (DIP), metacarpophalangeal (MCP) range of motion*
    - Wrist flexion and extension: *full range of motion intact*
  - Passive:
    - *Full range of motion intact*
    - Laxity / subluxation: *none*
- Function:
  - Pincer grip: *can grab a small coin out of examiner's grip*
  - Power grip: *5/5 power when squeezing examiner's finger with fist*
  - Fine motor: *can write their name and undo a shirt button*

Special tests

- Tinel's test: *no paraesthesia elicited*
- Phalen's test: *onset of pain within 30 seconds*
- Durkan's test: *onset of pain and paraesthesia in the median nerve distribution within 30 seconds*
- Finkelstein's test: *no pain along distal radius / negative test*

Investigations

BBMI-O: Bedside, **B**loods, **M**icrobiology, **I**maging and **O**ther

Investigation	Rationale
Bedside	
Bloods	
FBC, CRP	Looking for infection; inflammatory response
U&Es and creatinine	Assessing for electrolyte imbalances and renal function
CMP	Assessing calcium and nutrient levels
Uric acid	Looking for gout
ESR, RF	Looking for rheumatoid / acute phase reactants
Microbiology	
Imaging	
X-ray wrist and hand	Looking for bone pathologies, changes
MRI	Looking for soft tissue pathologies and changes, avascular necrosis, lesions causing compression
Other	
Electrodiagnostic testing: nerve conduction studies, EMG	Looking for neurological aetiologies

Diagnosis

Carpal tunnel syndrome

A patient with positive Phalen's and Durkan's test with a history of hand overuse, together with median nerve symptoms, is suspicious of carpal tunnel syndrome.

Discussion

Carpal tunnel syndrome is a clinical diagnosis:
- Pathology: not necessary in diagnosis (unless indicated pre-operatively in context of significant comorbidity)
- Imaging: not necessary in diagnosis
- Nerve conduction study, electromyogram (EMG): not necessary in diagnosis; may be performed in context of work compensation / legal issues.

Management

Non-operative

- Symptom management:
  - Simple analgesia (NSAIDs)
  - Corticosteroid injection
  - Wrist splints (usually at night)
- Lifestyle modification:
  - Activity modification
  - Risk factor modification

Operative

- Open carpal tunnel release:
  - Transverse carpal ligament is fully released in theatre

Other differential diagnoses

- Amyloidosis
- Reactive arthritis (e.g. Reiter's syndrome)
- Osteoarthritis
- Ulnar neuropathy
- Tenosynovitis (e.g. de Quervain syndrome)
- Other sites of median nerve compression
- Myelopathy

Station 35 **Headache**

An 18-year-old woman presents to the GP with a headache.

Tasks

1 Take a history
2 Perform a targeted examination
3 Describe appropriate investigations
4 Formulate a management plan

Differential diagnoses (VIITAMINC)

Vascular:
- Subarachnoid haemorrhage
- Sagittal sinus thrombosis
- Temporal arteritis

Infective:
- Meningitis
- Encephalitis
- Tropical illness

Inflammatory:
- Acute sinusitis
- Cluster headache
- Glaucoma

Trauma:
- Cervical spondylosis

Autoimmune

Metabolic

Iatrogenic:
- Rebound headache – medication overuse

Neoplastic:
- Intracranial mass causing raised intracranial pressure (ICP)

Congenital

Other:
- Migraine
- Tension headache
- Benign intracranial hypertension

Before starting

Establish rapport:
- Introduce yourself
- Obtain consent to take a history and examine the patient
- Expose the patient adequately

Confirm patient details:
- Name   *Bella Thomas*
- Age   *18 years*
- Occupation   *Student*

History

Ask about the pain (SOCRATES)

- **S**ite: *front of the head, involving behind the eyes*
- **O**nset: *sudden*
- **C**haracter: *pulsating*
- **R**adiation: *nil*
- **A**ssociated symptoms: *photophobia / phonophobia, nausea / vomiting*
- **T**ime: *started this morning*
- **E**xacerbating / relieving: *worse in bright rooms and loud noises, better when lying down in a dark room*
- **S**everity: *10/10*

Headache history

- Quality of the headache: *throbbing / tight sensation*
- Location of the headache: *over the frontal area*
- Severity and length: *as above; sudden, but not that severe*
- Is there any warning that the headache is about to come on (e.g. flashing lights, zigzag lines in vision): *yes, had flashing of vision just before the headache came on*

- Associated photophobia: *yes*
- Drowsiness or nausea: *no*
- Associated watering eye: *no*
- Recent consumption of alcohol: *yesterday, though only 2 drinks*

Past medical history and family history

- *No history of headaches*
- *Painful menstruation*
- *Mother has migraines, father has hypertension*

Drug history and allergies

- *Combined oral contraceptive pill*
- *NKDA*

Social history

- Smoking history: *2 pack-years*
- Alcohol and drugs history: *social drinker, binge drinking most weekends; nil illicit drugs*

Examination

General inspection (ABCD-V)

- **A**ppearance: *patient looks in pain*
- **B**ody habitus: *overweight, BMI 28*
- **C**ognition: *conscious and oriented*
- **D**evices / **D**rugs: *nil*
- **V**itals: *within normal limits*

Neurological examination

- Cranial nerves: *normal, mild photophobia when looking at CN II; pupils equal and reactive to light; symmetrical facial movements and intact sensation bilaterally*
- Inspection: *no abnormalities seen*
- Power / tone: *normal power and tone bilaterally*
- Sensation: *normal globally*
- Reflexes: *normal*

Investigations

BBMI-O: Bedside, **B**loods, **M**icrobiology, **I**maging and **O**ther

Investigation	Rationale
Bedside	
Bloods	
FBC	Looking for infection and anaemia
CRP	Looking for infection
ESR	Inflammatory marker
LFTs	Assess medication toxicity
U&Es and creatinine	Looking for electrolyte imbalances (particularly calcium) and renal injury
Blood cultures	Looking for a source of infection, if concerned for sepsis, meningitis, encephalitis
Microbiology	
Imaging	
CT / MRI brain	Looking for cranial pathology (e.g. tumour, raised ICP)
Other	
Lumbar puncture ± opening pressure	CSF fluid MCS and cell count; opening pressure looking for raised CSF

Diagnosis

Common migraine with aura

A history of headaches associated with photophobia relieving with rest in a young patient is most likely migraine.

Management

Lifestyle

- Avoid triggers (**CHOCOLATE**): **Ch**eese, **O**ral contraceptive pill, **C**affeine, al**co**hol, **A**nxiety, **T**ravel / Movement, **E**xercise
- Adequate nutrition and fluids

Medical

- Analgesia: diclofenac
- Anti-emetics as required
- 5HT-antagonist (i.e. triptans, ergotamine)
- Beta-blocker (i.e. propranolol)

Other differential diagnoses

- Benign intracranial hypertension
- Tension type headache

Station 36 **Hearing loss**

A 45-year-old man presents to his GP with reports of unilateral decreased hearing over his left ear over the past 12 months.

Tasks

1 Take a history
2 Perform a targeted examination
3 Describe appropriate investigations
4 Formulate a management plan

Differential diagnoses (VIITAMINC)

Vascular:
- Aneurysm
- Stroke
- Intracranial haemorrhage

Infective

Inflammatory:
- Middle ear effusion
- Otosclerosis
- Cholesteatoma
- Ménière's disease

Trauma:
- Noise-induced trauma

Autoimmune:
- Multiple sclerosis

Metabolic

Iatrogenic

Neoplastic:
- Acoustic neuroma
- Meningioma
- Chordoma
- Chondrosarcoma

Congenital

Other

Before starting

Establish rapport:
- Introduce yourself
- Consent the patient: "I'll be asking you some questions regarding your symptoms, and then I will need to perform a neurological exam and also some tests of your hearing"
- Expose the patient: as required

Confirm patient details:
- Name   *Andrzej Kowalski*
- Age   *45 years*
- Occupation *Builder*

History

History of presenting complaint

- Onset: *insidious, over the last year*

- Cochlear nerve symptoms:
  - *Increasing intermittent dizziness*
  - *Increasing prevalence of ipsilateral tinnitus*
  - *Difficulty localising sounds*
  - *Some episodic ipsilateral headaches*
- Vestibular nerve symptoms:
  - *Slight unsteadiness on ambulation which fluctuates*
  - *No overt vertigo, but can be brought on by head tilting*
- Trigeminal nerve symptoms:
  - *Facial paraesthesia*
- Facial nerve symptoms:
  - *Possible decreased taste*
  - *Possible increased lacrimation*
- Other symptoms:
  - *Denies loss of consciousness, change in cognition or memory*

- *Denies facial droop, slurred speech, weakness of body or limbs*
- Trauma: *none; no recent surgery*
- Constitutional symptoms: *none*

Past medical history and family history

- *Nil significant past medical history*
- *No family history*

Drug history and allergies

- *Nil*
- *NKDA*

Social history

- Smoking history: *non-smoker*
- Alcohol and drugs history: *non-drinker, nil illicit drugs*
- *Works in building and maintaining telecommunication towers*

Examination

General inspection (ABCD-V)

- **A**ppearance: *patient looks comfortable*
- **B**ody habitus: *normal, BMI 22*
- **C**ognition: *patient is conscious and oriented*
- **D**evices / **D**rugs: *nil*
- **V**itals: *all within normal limits*

Ear examination

- General inspection:
  - Facial appearance: *no droop or asymmetry*
  - Ears (pinnae): *no scars, signs of infection, trauma, erythema or swelling*
- Palpation:
  - *No facial or external auricular abnormalities palpated*
  - *No pain on palpation over the mastoid and external auricle*
- Movement:
  - Proprioception: *Romberg's test negative*
  - Vertigo: *Hallpike test negative*
- Neurology:
  - Cranial nerve exam (excluding CN VIII)
    - *Slight hyperaesthesia over the left face (CN V)*

Special tests

- Otoscopy:
  - Canal: *no discharge, swelling, erythema or foreign body*
  - Tympanic membrane: *normal colour, light reflex noted; no erythema, bulge, scarring or perforation*
- Weber's test: *sensorineural deafness positive: sound is decreased in the affected ear*
- Rinne's test: *sensorineural deafness positive: both air and bone reduced equally*

Investigations

BBMI-O: Bedside, **B**loods, **M**icrobiology, **I**maging and **O**ther

Investigation	Rationale
Bedside	
Bloods	
FBC	For preoperative work-up – look for anaemia
U&Es and creatinine	Assess renal function
Microbiology	
Imaging	
MRI	Assessing for intracranial mass / cause for hearing loss
Other	
Audiometry	Assess the extent and type of hearing loss

Diagnosis

Acoustic neuroma

A patient with insidious onset of the triad of unilateral hearing loss, tinnitus and dizziness requires investigation for acoustic neuroma.

Management

Non-operative

- Observation
  - Small tumours with minimal symptoms, with no enlargement on serial scanning
- Radiation therapy
  - Stereotactic radiosurgery
  - Stereotactic radiotherapy

Operative

- Surgical resection
  - Retromastoid suboccipital
  - Translabyrinthine
  - Middle fossa

Other differential diagnoses

- Meningioma
- Ménière's disease

Station 37 **Hypertension**

A 60-year-old man has been sent into your department by his local pharmacy after a free blood pressure reading yielded a systolic pressure of 190mmHg.

Tasks

1 Take a history
2 Perform a targeted examination

3 Describe appropriate investigations
4 Formulate a management plan

Differential diagnosis (VIITAMINC)

Vascular:
- Hypertension
- Left ventricular failure
- Aortic dissection
- Hypertensive encephalopathy
- Malignant hypertension

Infective

Inflammatory

Trauma

Autoimmune

Metabolic:
- Thyroid dysfunction
- Hyperparathyroidism
- Primary aldosteronism
- Kidney dysfunction

Iatrogenic:
- Corticosteroid use
- Atypical antipsychotic use

Neoplastic:
- Phaeochromocytoma

Congenital

Other

Before starting

Establish rapport:
- Introduce yourself
- Consent the patient: "I'll be asking you some questions regarding your symptoms, and then I will need to perform a full body examination"
- Expose the patient: when physical examination is required, it will require shirt/vest to be taken off

Patient profile:
- Name   *Harry Milligan*
- Age   *60 years*
- Occupation   *Office worker*

History

History of presenting complaint

- *Denies chest pain, dizziness, malaise*

- *Reports occasional palpitations and dyspnoea, but none currently*
- *Reports some dysphagia: chokes easily on food if not concentrating*
- *Change in bowel habits: loose bowels for several months*
- *Intolerance to hot/cold weather: noticed has been feeling overly hot, easily sweats and needs the air conditioning on every day*
- *Constitutional symptoms: no night sweats or fatigue; has lost 4kg in the past few months*

Past medical history and family history

- *Comorbidities: paroxysmal atrial fibrillation, type 2 diabetes mellitus – hard to control blood glucose recently*
- *Denies previous surgery or radiation to neck; denies special exposure to iodine*
- *Family history: positive for thyroid disease*

Drug history and allergies

- *Metformin, trialling gliclazide*
- *NKDA*

Social history

- *Office worker*
- *Current smoker, 14 per day*
- *Patient does not drink alcohol*

Examination

General inspection: (ABCD-V)

- **A**ppearance: *patient is inappropriately dressed for the weather and looking sweaty despite the lack of clothing*
- **B**ody habitus: *normal, BMI 20*
- **C**ognition: *patient is conscious and oriented*
- **D**evices / **D**rugs: *no*
- **V**itals: *BP 190/100mmHg, HR 110bpm and regular; other vital signs are within normal range*

Thyroid examination

- Inspection:
  - Skin: *warm and sweaty*
  - Eyes: *exophthalmos, lid retraction present*

- Chest: *nil gynaecomastia*
- Lower limbs: *nil pretibial myxoedema*
- Neck: *no pre-existing surgical scars around neck*
- Goitre: *rises when patient swallows*
- Palpation:
  - Goitre: *enlarged in size, uniform in shape with a regular isthmus, firm consistency, and non-tender*
  - Thrill (may be present and palpable in thyrotoxicosis): *not present in this case*
  - Auscultation (for a bruit): *negative*
  - Percussion (can help ascertain if the goitre extends retrosternally): *no extension*
  - Limb reflexes: *brisk*
- Movement:
  - Lid lag: *present as patient's eyes look from upper to lower visual fields*
  - Pemberton's sign: *not present*
  - Upper limb proximal myopathy: *negative*
  - Tremor: *present*
  - Lower limb proximal myopathy: *positive*

Investigations

BBMI-O: Bedside, **B**loods, **M**icrobiology, **I**maging and **O**ther

Investigation	Rationale
Bedside	
Bloods	
FBC / U&Es and creatinine	Baseline / pre-operative work-up
TSH, free T_3 and T_4	Assess renal function
LDL and HDL	Monitoring levels as they change post treatment for hyperthyroidism
Microbiology	
Imaging	
Thyroid ultrasound	Assesses for nodules
Thyroid isotope scan	Distinguish between Graves' disease and multinodular goitre
Bone scan	Assessing for bone metastasis
Other	

Diagnosis

Hyperthyroidism

This patient presents with several signs and symptoms of hyperthyroidism, which must be investigated.

Management

Non-operative (can be used in conjunction with operative)
- Thionamides:
  - Preferable for patients with or at risk for significant symptoms; medical management to achieve a rapid euthyroid status
- Radio-iodine ablation:
  - Patients with tolerable symptoms
  - Contraindicated in pregnancy and lactation
  - Administered orally

Operative

- Thyroidectomy:
  - Patients with severe hyperthyroidism and a large goitre
- Also for patients unable to take thionamides or radio-iodine therapy
- Pre- and postoperative vocal cord check required
- Require thyroid replacement therapy once levels return to normal postoperatively
- Blood pressure expected to decrease postoperatively
- Weight gain expected postoperatively

Other differential diagnoses

- Primary hypertension
- Hypothyroidism
- Thyroiditis

Station 38 **Incontinence**

A 60-year-old woman, G3P4, presents to your GP practice seeking advice as she reports the loss of control of her bladder when undergoing everyday activities.

Tasks

1 Take a history
2 Describe the steps to an appropriate pelvic examination

3 Describe appropriate investigations
4 Formulate a management plan

Differential diagnoses (VIITAMINC)

Vascular:
- Stroke

Infective:
- Urinary tract infection

Inflammatory:
- Urogenital fistula

Trauma:
- Stress incontinence

Autoimmune

Metabolic:
- Genitourinary syndrome of menopause / vaginal atrophy

Iatrogenic

Neoplastic:
- Malignancy

Congenital

Other:
- Urge incontinence
- Overflow incontinence:
  - Detrusor underactivity
  - Bladder outlet obstruction
- Parkinson's disease

Before starting

Establish rapport:
- Introduce yourself
- Consent the patient: "I'll be asking you some questions regarding your symptoms and some details about your past medical history; I'll also need to examine your pelvic and groin region, with your permission"
- Exposure: explain to the patient that you will need to do a pelvic examination and consider need for chaperone

Confirm patient details:
- Name   *Michelle Llewellyn*
- Age   *60 years*
- Occupation   *Unemployed*

History

History of presenting complaint
- Onset: *with coughing, sneezing and laughing over the last 12 months*
- Frequency: *daily*
- Severity: *requiring daily pad use to manage incontinence*
- Associated symptoms:
  - *Denies frequency, nocturia, hesitancy, decreased stream, incomplete voiding, polyuria, dysuria, froth in urine, renal colic, abdominal pain, fever*
- Description of stools: *denies melaena or per rectal bleed*
- Trauma: *none; no recent surgery*
- Constitutional symptoms: *none*

Obstetric history

- G3P4
- Three normal vaginal deliveries (one with twins)

Past medical history and family history

- Depression, type 2 diabetes mellitus (T2DM; diet-managed), obesity
- Hysterectomy for postpartum haemorrhage 14 years ago
- Mother had T2DM, chronic obstructive pulmonary disease

Drug history and allergies

- Nil
- NKDA

Social history

- Smoking history: 10 pack-years
- Alcohol and drugs history: social drinker, nil illicit drugs
- Home with family; caregiver for her family
- Daily caffeine intake

Examination

General inspection (ABCD-V)

- **A**ppearance: patient looks comfortable
- **B**ody habitus: overweight, BMI 28

- **C**ognition: patient is conscious and oriented
- **D**evices / **D**rugs: nil
- **V**itals: BP 130/70mmHg, HR 70bpm and regular; afebrile

Pelvic examination

The patient will rest in a lithotomy position:
- General inspection:
  - Note external perineal anatomy
  - Vaginal discharge: none
  - Rash or erythema: none
  - Vaginal atrophy: present
  - With the patient bearing down:
    - Cystocele: absent
    - Uterine prolapse: absent
- Palpation:
  - Bimanual palpation of the uterus / vaginal wall:
    - Vaginal bulge: absent
    - Urethral abnormality: absent
    - Genitourinary fistula: absent
    - Urethral diverticulum: absent
- Special tests:
  - Urethral mobility (required as pre-operative assessment for mid-urethral sling surgery) with a lubricated Q-tip
  - Bladder stress test:
    - Confirms diagnosis of stress incontinence

Investigations

BBMI-O: Bedside, **B**loods, **M**icrobiology, **I**maging and **O**ther

Investigation	Rationale
Bedside	
Bloods	
FBC, U&Es and creatinine, CRP	Only as pre-operative work-up
Microbiology	
Urine MCS	Assess for infective causes of incontinence
Imaging	
Other	

Diagnosis

Stress urinary incontinence

Management

Non-operative

- Pelvic floor strengthening: through physiotherapy exercises
- Lifestyle modification: diet, weight loss, avoiding constipation, smoking cessation
- Topical vaginal oestrogen
- Pessaries

Operative

For patients with no success on non-operative management or pessaries:
- Mid-urethral sling: a synthetic mesh is placed tension-free at the level of the mid-urethra

Other differential diagnoses

- Urinary tract infection
- Urge incontinence
- Overflow incontinence

Station 39 **Jaundice**

A 48-year-old woman presents to the emergency department with acute abdominal pain, nausea and vomiting, and yellow discolouration of the skin.

Tasks

1 Take a history
2 Perform a targeted examination
3 Describe appropriate investigations
4 Formulate a management plan

Differential diagnoses (VIITAMINC)

Vascular

Infective:
- Ascending cholangitis
- Hepatitis

Inflammatory:
- Steatohepatitis
- Cholelithiasis
- Choledocholithiasis
- Haemolytic anaemia

Trauma

Autoimmune

Metabolic:
- End-stage liver disease
- Gilbert's syndrome
- Haemochromatosis

Iatrogenic:
- Postoperative strictures
- Drug- and toxin-induced

Neoplastic:
- Pancreatic malignancy
- Cholangiocarcinoma

Congenital

Other:
- Pregnancy (HELLP syndrome)

Before starting

Establish rapport:
- Introduce yourself
- Consent the patient: "I'll be asking you some questions regarding your symptoms and also some details about your past medical history; later I will also be examining your abdomen"
- Expose the patient: when physical examination is required, it will require top / vest to be taken off; consider the need for a chaperone

Confirm patient details:
- Name   *Elizabeth Moore*
- Age   *48 years*
- Occupation   *Lawyer*

History

Pain history (SOCRATES)

- **S**ite: *right abdomen*
- **O**nset: *sudden, 1 hour after lunch*
- **C**haracter: *sharp, rapid rise to maximal intensity; comes and goes*
- **R**adiation: *travels around the right ribs to the back*
- **A**ssociated symptoms: *initial nausea and vomiting; denies fevers; denies chest pain or shortness of breath*
- **T**ime / duration: *each episode lasts half an hour*
- **E**xacerbating / relieving factors: *unrelated to position; self-limiting episodes*
- **S**everity: *severe, debilitating during episodes*

History of presenting complaint

- Previous episodes: *similar pain 3 months back, lesser intensity, self-resolved*
- *Denies anorexia*
- *Denies recent travel*
- *Denies urinary symptoms*
- *Denies bowel changes, per rectal bleed, melaena*
- *Denies constitutional symptoms*

Past medical history and family history

- *Hypercholesterolaemia*
- Surgical history: *appendicectomy*
- *Nil family history*

Drug history and allergies

- *Nil*
- *NKDA*

Social history

- Smoking history: *non-smoker*
- Alcohol and drugs history: *social drinker, nil illicit drugs*

Examination

General inspection (ABCD-V)

- **A**ppearance: *patient appears in pain*
- **B**ody habitus: *overweight, BMI 27*
- **C**ognition: *patient is conscious and oriented*
- **D**evices / **D**rugs: *no*
- **V**itals: *BP 140/90mmHg, HR 95bpm and regular; other vital signs are within normal range*

Gastrointestinal examination

- Inspection:
  - Skin: *jaundice, scleral icterus; no spider naevi (liver disease) or petechiae (alcoholism)*
  - Hands: *no palmar erythema (liver disease)*
  - Abdomen:
    - *No distension (ascites, liver disease)*
    - *No caput medusae (liver disease)*
    - *Previous laparoscopic appendicectomy scar visible*
- Palpation:
  - *Soft abdomen; no guarding or signs of peritonism*
  - *Right upper quadrant (RUQ) tenderness*
  - *Murphy's positive*
  - *No masses palpable; no organomegaly*
- Percussion:
  - *Percussion resonant*
- Auscultation:
  - *Normal bowel sounds*

Investigations

BBMI-O: Bedside, **B**loods, **M**icrobiology, **I**maging and **O**ther

Investigation	Rationale
Bedside	
ECG	Rule out cardiac disease
Bloods	
FBC, CRP	Assessing infection and inflammatory markers
U&Es and creatinine	Assessing renal function
LFTs, coagulation profile	Assessing liver function (especially ALP and GGT indicating an obstructive picture)
Conjugated, unconjugated bilirubin	Assessing for the cause of hyperbilirubinaemia
Lipase	Assessing for associated pancreatitis
Beta-hCG	Ensure not pregnancy related

Investigation	Rationale
Microbiology	
▨ Urine MCS	▨ Rule out urinary tract infection
Imaging	
▨ Abdominal US	▨ Evaluate liver, gallbladder, biliary tree and pancreas
▨ MRCP	▨ Better visualise the biliary tree once choledocholithiasis seen on ultrasound
Other	
▨ Colonoscopy ± biopsies	▨ Looking for areas of thickened bowel wall, inflamed bowel wall; positive biopsies would be indicative of malignancy

Diagnosis

Choledocholithiasis

A patient with jaundice, RUQ pain and a positive Murphy's sign is highly suggestive of biliary colic.

The gold standard investigation to confirm choledocholithiasis is a RUQ US with reference to LFTs.

Management

- ▨ Intravenous antibiotics:
  - If signs or symptoms of cholecystitis
- ▨ Endoscopic retrograde cholangiopancreatography (ERCP):
  - To retrieve stone in common bile duct
- ▨ Cholecystectomy:
  - Laparoscopic or open
  - Intraoperative cholangiogram assesses for retained stones in biliary tree

- If stone seen on cholangiogram:
  - ▸ Intraoperative common bile duct exploration, or
  - ▸ Intraoperative ERCP, or
  - ▸ Postoperative ERCP

Other differential diagnoses

- ▨ Acute cholangitis
- ▨ Pancreatic malignancy

Station 40 **Joint pain and deformity**

A 70-year-old man presents to your clinic with a bowed leg, unilateral knee pain and increasing difficulty in weight-bearing.

Tasks

1 Take a history
2 Perform a targeted examination

3 Describe appropriate investigations
4 Formulate a management plan

Differential diagnosis (VIITAMINC)

Vascular:
- Deep vein thrombosis

Infective:
- Septic arthritis
- Osteoarthritis of knee / hip

Inflammatory:
- Sciatica
- Bursitis

Trauma:
- Fracture
- Ligament tears
- Meniscal tears

- Muscle sprain

Autoimmune:
- Rheumatoid arthritis

Metabolic:
- Rickets

Iatrogenic

Neoplastic

Congenital:
- Skeletal dysplasia
- Asymmetric growth

Other

Before starting

Establish rapport:
- Introduce yourself
- Consent the patient: "I'll be asking you some questions regarding your knee pain, then I will need you to remove your bottom clothing, so we can have a look at your legs and have you do some movements, would that be OK?"
- Expose the patient: during physical examination; both lower legs need to be exposed for assessment and comparison; the patient can keep their underwear on for comfort, provided the hips can be grossly assessed

Confirm patient details:
- Name   *Jerry James*
- Age   *70 years*
- Occupation   *Retired, though construction worker in the past*

History

Pain history (SOCRATES)
- **S**ite: *entire left knee joint*
- **O**nset: *during ambulation and weight-bearing on affected joint*
- **C**haracter: *sharp, locking and catching sensations; stiffness; joint can feel unstable*
- **R**adiation: *localised to the knee*
- **A**ssociated symptoms: *swelling in knee*
- **T**ime / duration: *has been an issue for the past 3 years*

Exacerbating / relieving factors: *pain is relieved by rest; exacerbated by ambulation*

Severity: *intense pain after 5 minutes of walking which impedes further ambulation*

Musculoskeletal and rheumatological history

- Preceding trauma to the region: *no*
- Other joint involvement: *no*
- Constitutional symptoms: *no*
- Neurological symptoms: *no*
- Skin changes: *no*

Past medical history and family history

- *Type 2 diabetes mellitus, hypertension*
- *Nil family history*

Drug history and allergies

- *Perindopril, metformin*
- *NKDA*

Social history

- Smoking history: *non-smoker*
- Alcohol and drugs history: *non-drinker, nil illicit drugs*

Examination

General inspection (ABCD-V)

- **A**ppearance: *patient looks comfortable*
- **B**ody habitus: *overweight, BMI 28*
- **C**ognition: *patient is conscious and oriented*
- **D**evices / **D**rugs: *nil*
- **V**itals: *BP 130/70mmHg, HR 70bpm and regular; afebrile*

Knee examination

- Inspection:
  - Have the patient standing for the inspection component to assess while weight-bearing:
    - Gait: *mild limp noted, favouring the right leg*
    - Deformity: *varus deformity present*
  - Lie the patient down:
    - Skin: *no*
    - Swelling: *no*
  - Muscle bulk: *left thigh looks smaller compared with right*
- Palpation:
  - Masses: *no*
  - Temperature: *normal*
  - Tenderness: *tender along joint line of the knee (best elicited with the knee in slight flexion)*
  - Effusion: *no*
  - Muscle bulk: *moderate atrophy, left worse than right*
- Movement:
  - Active – begin with the side least affected:
    - Limited movement bilaterally, left worse than right
    - Patellar subluxation: *negative*
    - Feel for crepitus (in active or passive movement): *present*
  - Passive – begin with the side least affected:
    - Flexion, extension: *Full ROM*
    - Medial and lateral collateral ligaments: *normal*
    - McMurray's test: *normal*
    - Lachman test: *normal*
    - Patellar apprehension test: *normal*
    - Apley's grind test: *unable to perform due to the reduced range of movement*

Investigations

BBMI-O: Bedside, **B**loods, **M**icrobiology, **I**maging and **O**ther

Investigation	Rationale
Bedside	
Bloods	
FBC, U&Es and creatinine, coagulation profile	As part of preoperative work-up if pursuing with surgical management
CMP, vitamin D	Assessing bone health; osteoporosis screen

Investigation	Rationale
◼ CRP, ESR	◼ Screening for active infection or inflammation (e.g. rheumatoid arthritis flare), which are contraindications for operative management
Microbiology	
Imaging	
◼ Knee X-ray	◼ Confirms diagnosis and evaluates the extent of degenerative changes: loss of joint space, osteophytes, subchondral sclerosis, subchondral cysts
◼ MRI	◼ To evaluate menisci and ligaments, if suspicious of soft tissue cause
Other	

Diagnosis

Degenerative osteoarthritis

A relatively benign history with a normal passive musculoskeletal examination suggests that pain is the main cause of the patient's limited movement, and osteoarthritis is most likely.

Management

Non-operative

◼ Symptom management (first-line treatment):
  • Simple analgesia (NSAIDs)
  • Intra-articular steroid injection
◼ Lifestyle modification:
  • Activity modification
  • Risk factor modification – weight loss, diet
◼ Physiotherapy, exercise programmes:
  • Quadriceps strengthening

Operative

If non-operative management has failed:
◼ Arthroplasty:
  • Unicompartmental knee replacement: when arthritic changes are isolated to one compartment of the knee
  • Total knee replacement

The patient is to begin weight-bearing and immediate physiotherapy with optimal range of movement postoperative day 1.

Other differential diagnoses

◼ Rheumatoid arthritis
◼ Meniscal injury
◼ Anterior cruciate ligament injuries
◼ Medial collateral ligament (MCL) injuries
◼ Lateral collateral ligament (LCL) injuries

Station 41 **Leg pain**

An elderly woman presents to the emergency department with a 3-week history of left leg pain.

Tasks

1 Take a history
2 Perform a targeted examination
3 Describe appropriate investigations
4 Formulate a management plan

Differential diagnoses (VIITAMINC)

Vascular:
- Peripheral vascular disease
- Vasculitic neuropathy
- Thrombophlebitis
- Arterial or venous ulcers
- Deep or superficial venous thrombosis

Infective:
- Cellulitis
- Septic arthritis
- Hepatitis

Inflammatory:
- Transient synovitis
- Lymphadenitis
- Bursitis

Trauma:
- Haematoma
- Wound, e.g. laceration, bullet wound
- Fracture
- Sciatica
- Compartment syndrome
- Ligamentous or muscle tear or strain
- Ruptured Baker's cyst

Allergy/**A**utoimmune:
- Arthritis in joints
- Monoclonal gammopathy

Metabolic:
- Muscle cramping

- Diabetic neuropathy

Idiopathic/**I**atrogenic:
- Myositis
- Lumbar canal stenosis
- Perthe's disease
- Patellofemoral pain syndrome
- Slipped capital femoral epiphysis/slipped upper femoral epiphysis (SUFE)
- Osgood–Schlatter disease
- Complex regional pain syndrome
- Medications: statins, diuretics, some antihypertensives, antipsychotics
- Deficiencies: chronic B_{12} deficiency resulting in a spastic neuropathy

Neoplastic:
- Leukaemia
- Metastasis to lower limb bones from primary cancers in kidney, breast, prostate, lung and thyroid
- Primary muscular or bone tumour
- Paraproteinaemic neuropathy
- Paraneoplastic neuropathy

Congenital/**C**hromosomal:
- Cerebral palsy with spastic paralysis
- Femoral anteversion
- Hereditary spastic paraplegia

Before starting

Establish rapport:
- Introduce yourself
- Obtain consent to take a history and examine the patient
- Expose the patient: when physical examination is required

Confirm patient details:
- Name — *Beverly Hills*
- Age — *72 years*
- Occupation — *Retired florist*

History

History of presenting complaint (SOCRATES)

- **S**ite: *left lower back down to left foot*
- **O**nset: *last 4 days, progressively worsening, now unable to sit; started when bent over to pick up a box of clothes from the floor*
- **C**haracter: *sharp, burning pain similar to electric shock down the leg; associated with some pins and needles and numbness*
- **R**adiation: *pain starts from left back and radiates down the back of the left leg into the foot*
- **A**ssociated features: *associated with some calf tenderness but mainly just shooting pains; no swelling, fevers or loss of weight*
- **T**ime course: *as per onset; this is not the first time this pain has come on, though is the worst; usually lasts 2–5 days*
- **E**xacerbating and relieving factors: *worse on bending and sitting, improves on standing or lying still; paracetamol at home has not helped, where in the past this has improved the pain*
- **S**everity: *now unable to sit down; also having trouble sleeping and doing daily activities due to the pain*

Past medical history and family history

- *Osteoarthritis of knees, hypertension, chronic back pain*
- *Mother had osteoarthritis, father had heart attack at age 60 years*

Drug history and allergies

- *Ramipril, paracetamol*
- *NKDA*

Social history

- Smoking history: *10 pack-years*
- Alcohol and drugs history: *1–2 glasses of wine per day, nil illicit drugs*

Examination

General inspection (ABCD-V)

- **A**ppearance: *patient appears to be in pain, standing uncomfortably*
- **B**ody habitus: *obese, BMI 31*
- **C**ognition: *patient is conscious and oriented*
- **D**evices / **D**rugs: *no*
- **V**itals: *BP 140/90mmHg, HR 95bpm and regular; other vital signs are within normal range*

Lower limb examination

- Inspection:
  - Scars that may indicate past bypass surgery from vein harvest or healed ulcers: *no*
  - Lower limb hair loss and the shape of 'inverted champagne bottle' in peripheral vascular disease (PVD): *no*
  - Discoloration, e.g. erythema, may indicate infection; necrosis or pallor peripherally indicates poor arterial perfusion: *no*
  - Previous amputations of toes or limbs: *no*
  - Muscle wasting: *no*
- Palpation:
  - *Warm and equal bilaterally*
  - *No tenderness on hip / knee palpation*
  - Capillary refill: *2–3 seconds*
  - Pitting or non-pitting oedema: *no oedema*
  - Presence of arterial pulses: *palpable lower limb pulses, regular and strong*
  - Calf circumference: *equal bilaterally*
  - Muscle bulk: *slightly reduced on the left thigh in comparison with the right*
- Movement:
  - Hip flexion / extension / abduction / adduction: *reduced range due to pain on left, full range on right*
  - Knee flexion / extension / abduction / adduction: *full range bilaterally*
  - Ankle and foot flexion / extension / abduction / adduction: *full range bilaterally*
- Neurological examination:
  - Tone: *normal*

- Power: *5/5 power bilaterally throughout entire lower limb*
- Sensation: *mildly reduced sensation in the distribution of pain, posterior proximal leg moving down to the lateral aspect of the calf and foot*
- Reflexes: *slightly reduced in left knee in compared with right; ankle and Babinski normal*

- Special tests:
  - Buerger's test in bilateral lower limbs: *negative*
  - Straight leg raise: *elicits pain on left leg*
  - Lower back examination: *no overt abnormalities bilaterally; mild tenderness to palpate the lower left region; muscle bulk symmetrical; no change in sensation bilaterally*

Investigations

BBMI-O: Bedside, **B**loods, **M**icrobiology, **I**maging and **O**ther

Investigation	Rationale
Bedside	
Bloods	
FBC	Infection and anaemia
CRP	Acute marker of inflammation
ESR	Chronic inflammatory disease states e.g. rheumatoid arthritis
U&Es and creatinine	Renal disease
Glucose level and HbA1c	Diabetes and its control
Lipid profile	Increased cholesterol indicates higher risk for PVD
Creatinine kinase	Rhabdomyolysis
Microbiology	
Imaging	
X-ray of affected limb and foot	Osteomyelitis, fracture, bone tumour, arthritis
CT angiography of lower limbs	Severity of peripheral vascular disease, presence of aneurysm(s), soft tissue or bone tumour
MRI lower limbs	Soft tissue tumour, tendon injury
Other	
Arthrocentesis (aspiration) of synovial joint effusion, preferably under US guidance	Septic joint, gout or haemarthrosis
Muscle biopsy may be indicated if a myositis or neuropathy is considered	Myositis
Tissue core biopsy	Soft tissue sarcoma

Investigation	Rationale
▓ Bone biopsy	▓ Bone tumour
▓ Ankle-brachial index	▓ Looking for higher peripheral vascular resistance
▓ Nerve conduction studies / electromyography (EMG)	▓ Myositis

Diagnosis

Sciatica

A history of recent trauma, with a positive straight leg raise, is typical of sciatica.

Management

Medical

▓ Analgesia:
  ● Paracetamol ± ibuprofen
  ● Opioid medications for severe pain
  ● Neuropathic pain medications: gabapentin, tramadol, etc.
  ● Corticosteroid injection
  ● Nerve blocks
▓ Physiotherapy – to strengthen the back muscles and aid in managing the neuropathic pain
▓ Conservative measures including rest, heat and massage

Surgical

▓ Only reserved for severe cases involving neurological compromise (i.e. spinal cord compression) and chronic sciatica impacting life on a daily basis
▓ As a mainstay intervention; includes microdiscectomy and discectomy

Other differential diagnoses

▓ Compartment syndrome
▓ Ischaemic limbs
▓ Fractures
▓ Lumbar canal stenosis
▓ Soft tissue sarcoma
▓ Bone tumours
▓ Spastic muscle contractures

Station 42 **Leg ulcer**

A 75-year-old man presents to the GP with a leg ulcer.

Tasks

1 Take a history
2 Perform a targeted examination
3 Describe appropriate investigations
4 Formulate a management plan

Differential diagnoses (VIITAMINC)

Vascular:
- Peripheral venous / arterial insufficiency
- Vasculitis
- Thromboangiitis obliterans
- Microvascular occlusion disorders

Infective:
- Cellulitis
- Tuberculosis
- Syphilis

Inflammatory:
- Pyoderma gangrenosum

Trauma:
- Burns, direct trauma, postsurgical

Autoimmune

Metabolic

Iatrogenic

Neoplastic:
- Melanoma
- Squamous cell carcinoma (SCC)
- Basal cell carcinoma (BCC)

Congenital

Other:
- Pressure ulcer
- Spider / snake bite

Before starting

Establish rapport:
- Introduce yourself
- Obtain consent to take a history and examine the patient
- Expose the patient: as appropriate

Confirm patient details:
- Name   *Barry Stream*
- Age   *75 years*
- Occupation   *Retired electrician*

History

Ask about the pain (SOCRATES)

- **S**ite: *distal left lateral calf*

- **O**nset: *noticed 2 months ago, has been progressively growing and worsening; recently it has began to have 'gunk' around it and smell*
- **C**haracter: *painless ulcer*
- **R**adiation: *nil*
- **A**ssociated symptoms: *slightly warm around the ulcer*
- **T**ime: *first noticed after a cut occurred to the area; this progressively worsened and became a non-healing ulcer*
- **E**xacerbating / relieving: *strict dressing care had slightly improved it, though recently nothing*
- **S**everity: *2–4/10, no pain just worsening size and condition*

Ulcer differential specific history

- Pain: *yes, burning / prickling in the hands and ankles*

- Paraesthesia / anaesthesia: *noticed change / dulling in sensation in the hands to the wrist and feet to mid calves bilaterally*
- Urinary frequency / urgency / nocturia: *yes, has noticed increased frequency and nocturia in the last 2 years*
- Erectile dysfunction: *no*
- Diabetes mellitus: *yes, poorly controlled*
- Intermittent claudication: *no*
- Peripheral oedema, relieved with elevation of the limb: *no*

Past medical history and family history

- *Hypertension, hypercholesterolaemia, type 2 diabetes (T2DM; uncontrolled), chronic renal disease, heart attack (10 years ago, required a stent)*
- *Previous foot ulcer on the left heel 12 months ago, required debridement and antibiotics for a superimposed* Staphylococcus aureus *infection*
- *Amputation of the left 5th foot phalange as complication of diabetes*
- *Mother had T2DM, hypertension and died of a stroke at 88 years; father had hypertension, osteoarthritis and T2DM*

Drug history and allergies

- *Ramipril, atenolol, atorvastatin, clopidogrel and aspirin*
- *Metformin, insulin: basal / bolus regimen; failed dual metformin and sitagliptin*
- *NKDA*

Social history

- Smoking history: *60 pack-years*
- Alcohol and drugs history: *social drinker, binge drinking most weekends, nil illicit drugs*
- *Lives at home alone, requires home support two times per week*
- *Requires a 4-wheel frame*

Examination

General inspection (ABCD-V)

- **A**ppearance: *patient looks well*
- **B**ody habitus: *obese, BMI 33*
- **C**ognition: *conscious and oriented*
- **D**evices / **D**rugs: *nil*

- **V**itals: *BP 165/100mmHg, HR 89bpm; other vitals within normal limits; afebrile*

Lower limb examination

- Inspection:
  - *Skin is hairless and atrophied*
  - Ulcer:
    - Site: *lower left lateral calf, 8cm superior to the lateral malleolus*
    - Size: *4.5 × 6.5cm, 1cm depth*
    - Shape: *rhomboid*
    - Shade: *mildly erythematous*
    - Symmetry: *no*
    - Substance (discharge): *yes, moderate amount of purulent exudate; minor necrotic area at the inferior border*
    - Smell: *malodorous*
    - Sides (borders): *sloping*
    - Surrounding skin: *slightly warm to palpate, no obvious erythema, oedema or maceration*
    - Sensation: *anaesthesia over and around the ulcer*
    - Scaling: *no*
  - *No signs of infections, i.e. cellulitis, athlete's foot, present on the ulcer site or in between the toes*
  - *Mild varicosities on the legs bilaterally*
  - *Venous staining present on distal calves bilaterally*
  - *No obvious deformities, amputated 5th phalange of the foot*
  - *No muscle wasting*
  - Gait: *imbalance on walking, decreased speed and increased base of gait*
- Palpation:
  - Temperature: *feet are cold to palpate*
  - Capillary refill: *3–4 seconds*
  - Pulses: *impalpable dorsalis pedis and posterior tibial; strong popliteal and femoral*
  - *No peripheral oedema*
- Special tests:
  - 10g monofilament: *reduced to no sensation to mid calf bilaterally*
  - Vibration sensation (128Hz tuning fork): *distal phalanx of great toes negative sensation bilaterally, medial malleolus negative on left and positive on the right*

- Buerger's test (peripheral vascular disease): *normal*
- Ankle-brachial index: *normal*
- Ulcer probe: *1cm deep, unable to probe to bone*

Neurological examination

- Inspection: *mild quadriceps wasting bilaterally*
- Power / tone: *normal power and tone bilaterally*

- Reflexes: *normal*
- Sensation: *complete anaesthesia of the toes and medial aspect of the plantar foot bilaterally, reduced sensation (light touch, pain and temperature) up to the mid calf bilaterally*
- Proprioception: *0/3 movements on the big toe, 2/3 movements on the ankles bilaterally*

Investigations

BBMI-O: Bedside, **B**loods, **M**icrobiology, **I**maging and **O**ther

Investigation	Rationale
Bedside	
Bloods	
FBC	Looking for infection and anaemia
CRP	Looking for infection
U&Es and creatinine	Looking for electrolyte imbalances (particularly calcium) and renal function
HbA1c / Blood glucose levels	Looking for diabetes / glycaemic control
Vitamin B_{12}	Looking for B_{12} deficiency as cause for peripheral neuropathy
Blood cultures	Looking for a source of infection, if concerned for sepsis
Microbiology	
Swab MCS	Looking for infection, cultures and specificities
Imaging	
X-ray	Looking for depth of ulcer / possible extension to bone
Lower limb US ± Doppler	Looking for vessel patency and flow volumes
CT / MRI angiography	Looking for peripheral artery disease, osteomyelitis and depth of ulcer
Other	
Bone biopsy	Looking to diagnose osteomyelitis
Skin biopsy	Looking for malignancy or vasculitis

Diagnosis

Diabetic ulcer: peripheral neuropathy

A patient with extensive diabetic history and a non-healing ulcer is typical of diabetic ulcers.

Grading system: Wagner ulcer classification system

Grade	Lesion
0	No open lesions, may have associated cellulitis or deformity
1	Superficial ulcer (partial or full thickness)
2	Extension of ulcer to the ligaments / tendons / joint capsule / deep fascia, without osteomyelitis or abscess
3	Deep ulcer with osteomyelitis, abscess or joint sepsis
4	Localised gangrene
5	Extensive gangrene

Management

Lifestyle

- Weight loss, optimised diet, smoking cessation, alcohol intake reduction, adequate exercise
- Patient education (on diabetes and complications) is a multidisciplinary approach: GP, diabetes educator, endocrinologist, podiatrist
- Pressure offloading on pressure areas and wounds
- Dressing:
  - Dry sloughy and necrotic wounds (moisture donating): hydrogel, moistened saline gauze
  - Low–moderate exudate: hydrocolloid
  - Moderate–high exudate: polyurethane, alginates, foams

Medical

- Glycaemic control optimisation: metformin, insulin (basal ± bolus dosing, short- versus long-acting)

- Neuropathic pain: i.e. gabapentin, pregabalin
- Antibiotics (infected ulcer):
  - Mild–moderate infection: amoxycillin + clavulanate or cephalexin and metronidazole for 5–7 days
  - Severe: piperacillin and tazobactam
- Hyperbaric oxygen therapy / negative pressure wound therapy: chronic, non-healing ulcers

Surgical

- Debridement of the ulcer: necrotic, non-viable, sloughing and infected areas
- Peripheral artery revascularisation: percutaneous transluminal angioplasty, luminal stenting, arterial reconstruction
- Amputation: if revascularisation is contraindicated, septic patients and extensive necrosis

Other differential diagnoses

- Venous insufficiency ulcer
- Arterial insufficiency ulcer

Station 43 **Limb weakness**

An 80-year-old man presents to the emergency department with lower limb weakness.

Tasks

1 Take a history
2 Perform a targeted examination
3 Describe appropriate investigations
4 Formulate a management plan

Differential diagnoses (VIITAMINC)

Vascular:
- Severe peripheral vascular disease
- Intracerebral bleed (ischaemic or haemorrhagic)

Infection:
- Post-infective: Guillain–Barré syndrome
- Viral causes:
  - Flaccid paralysis, e.g. West Nile virus
  - Epstein–Barr (EBV) or influenza (generalised myopathy)
  - HIV (limb weakness, hyper-reflexia, hypertonia)
  - Human T-cell lymphotrophic virus: polyneuropathies, motor neurone disease, myasthenia gravis-like syndrome
- Bacterial causes:
  - Diphtheria: proximal muscle weakness of extremities progressing distally
  - *Clostridium botulinum*: symmetric descending paralysis
  - Tetanus (*Clostridium tetani*): muscle rigidity and spasms
- Tick paralysis

Inflammatory:
- Drug-induced or autoimmune-triggered myositis

Trauma:
- Compartment syndrome
- Spinal cord injury
- Cauda equina syndrome:
  - Compression of the spinal canal below the level of the conus medullaris

- Lacerations to nerves supplying lower limbs, i.e. foot drop from laceration of deep fibular nerve supplying tibialis anterior
- Spinal cord degeneration: nerve compression results in pain and weakness

Autoimmune:
- Multiple sclerosis (more common in females)
- Hypo- and hyperthyroidism
- Myasthenia gravis
- Systemic lupus erythematosus (SLE)

Metabolic:
- Hypophosphataemia
- Uraemia
- Thiamine deficiency
- B_{12} deficiency
- Hypokalaemia
- Carnitine deficiency
- Acid maltase deficiency
- Chronic liver disease
- Lead and mercury poisoning
- Glucocorticoid excess

Idiopathic / **I**atrogenic:
- Drug-induced myopathy: amiodarone, chloroquine, heroin, lithium, misoprostol, nitrofurantoin, vincristine, statins
- Amyotrophic lateral sclerosis

Neoplasia:
- Central nervous system tumour
- Paraneoplastic phenomena

Congenital:
- Progressive weakness:
  - Charcot–Marie–Tooth disease
  - Cerebral palsy (usually identified within first few years of life)
  - Myotonic dystrophy (Steinert's disease)
- Duchenne muscular dystrophy (DMD)
- Fascioscapulohumeral muscular dystrophy
- Limb-girdle muscular dystrophy
- Juvenile amyotrophic lateral sclerosis

Before starting

Establish rapport:
- Introduce yourself
- Obtain consent to take a history and examine the patient
- Expose the patient: when physical examination is required
- Explain to the patient that you may need to do a rectal examination and consider need for chaperone

Confirm patient details:
- Name — *Sam Green*
- Age — *80 years*
- Occupation — *Retired, previously army officer*

History

History of presenting complaint (SOCRATES)

- **S**ite:
  - Weakness: *unilateral weakness of the entire limb*
  - Any other muscles affected: *no*
- **O**nset:
  - Onset: *gradual initially, though last week has declined rapidly*
  - Identify what muscle or region became weak first, and if any other muscles have been affected: *spread from thighs down, now entire leg*
- **C**haracter:
  - Standing from sitting: *no*
  - Tripping when walking or has a foot drop: *yes, tripping when walking*
  - Urinary retention and faecal incontinence: *yes, over the last week has double incontinence*
  - Difficulty swallowing or breathing: *no*

- **R**adiation:
  - Progressive weakness in lower limbs or ascending weakness: *progressive weakness, proximal to distal*
- **A**ssociated features:
  - Dysphonia: *no*
  - Throbbing pain: *no*
  - Numbness or neuropathic pain: *yes, associated numbness and paraesthesia*
  - Fasciculations: *no*
  - Recent illness: *no*
  - Rashes: *no*
  - Arthritis or arthralgias: *no*
  - Any eye signs: *no*
  - Dysphagia or dysarthria: *no*
  - Back pain: *yes, lower back*
  - Systemic symptoms: *yes, for the last 6 months*
  - Other: *has noticed difficulty urinating and occasional spots of blood in the urine over the last 18 months*
- **T**ime course:
  - Helps to differentiate between acute and chronic: *first noticed 8 months ago, progressive decline since then; over the last week has become debilitating*
  - Ask if symptoms wax and wane: *no*
- **E**xacerbating and relieving factors: *worse on movement, no complete improvement even at rest*
- **S**everity:
  - How is this affecting their life: *unable to perform activities around the house, such as gardening, cleaning and walking due to pain and weakness*
  - Ask specifically:
    - How long they could walk for before becoming weak: *0.5km*
    - Are they able to put their arms above their head: *yes*
    - Do they have progressive dysphagia: *no*

▷ Do they find repetitive motion tires their muscles out to the point of being unable to use them: *no*

Past medical history and family history

▦ *Hypertension, type 2 diabetes mellitus, arthritis*
▦ *Father had prostate cancer, mother died from a stroke at 85 years*

Drug history and allergies

▦ *Perindopril, metformin, paracetamol, ibuprofen*
▦ *NKDA*

Social history

▦ Smoking history: *non-smoker*
▦ Alcohol and drugs history: *3 beers per day, nil illicit drugs*

Examination

General inspection (ABCD-V)

▦ **A**ppearance: *patient looks comfortable*
▦ **B**ody habitus: *overweight, BMI 28*
▦ **C**ognition: *patient is conscious and oriented*
▦ **D**evices/**D**rugs: *nil*
▦ **V**itals: *BP 130/70mmHg, HR 70bpm and regular; afebrile*

Lower limb examination

▦ Inspection:
  ● Rashes: *no*
  ● Muscle wasting: *yes, left thigh in comparison with right*
  ● Bruising or petechiae: *some scattered bruises on lower limbs*
  ● Obvious deformity: *no*
  ● Foot ulcerations on base of feet: *no*
  ● Colour: *normal skin colour*
  ● Myxoedema: *no*
▦ Palpation:
  ● Oedema: *no*
  ● *Warm bilaterally*
  ● Arterial pulses: *normal*
  ● Capillary refill: *normal, <2 seconds*
  ● Masses: *no*
  ● Back: *tenderness on palpation at the level of L4/5, no obvious deformities, some wasting of the back muscles on the left*
▦ Movement:
  ● Tone: *normal*
  ● Power: *reduced on left; hip flexion/extension 3+/5, knee flexion/extension 3+/5, ankle flexion/extension 4–/5; right side normal 5/5 throughout*

Neurological examination

▦ Tone: *normal*
▦ Movement: *limited on left side due to pain*
▦ Sensation: *reduced on left in L4–S1 dermatomes*
▦ Reflexes: *hyper-reflexia of the knee and ankle, Babinski normal*
▦ Anal tone: *reduced*

Investigations

BBMI-O: Bedside, **B**loods, **M**icrobiology, **I**maging and **O**ther

Investigation	Rationale
Bedside	
Bloods	
▦ FBC	▦ Infection, inflammation, anaemia
▦ CRP	▦ Acute marker of inflammation
▦ U&Es and creatinine	▦ Renal disease
▦ ESR	▦ Chronic inflammatory disease
▦ Glucose level and HbA1c	▦ Diabetes and its control

Investigation	Rationale
Creatinine kinase	Muscle atrophy
Anti-endomysial and anti-AGA Ab	Myositis (antibodies to nerve cells)
Anti-acetylcholine receptor Ab	Myasthenia gravis
TFTs	Hypo- or hyperthyroidism
• Anti-TTG and anti-TSH Ab	• Progress onto these blood tests if TFTs are abnormal
Chromosomal analysis	If suspecting a genetic disorder, such as DMD

Microbiology

Nasopharyngeal aspirate	Influenza or EBV
Muscle biopsy (after an EMG)	Myositis / dermatomyositis
24-hour urine heavy metal titres – if history of lead or mercury exposure	Heavy metal toxicity

Imaging

X-ray to identify underlying fractures if suspecting trauma, or to investigate limbs or feet that are misaligned	Charcot foot in diabetics, or missed fracture causing pain and weakness (e.g. fractured neck of femur in elderly)
CT spine	More sensitive for spinal fracture causing spinal cord or nerve compression
CT angiography of lower limbs	Peripheral vascular disease or aneurysm
MRI	If suspecting a mass in the spine or lower limbs, or herniated disc, causing compressive symptoms; can also show inflammation within the muscle belly (myositis) but not diagnostic

Other

EMG and nerve conduction studies	Helps determine intrinsic neuropathy, myasthenia gravis or myopathy
Muscle biopsy	If considering myositis or muscular dystrophy
Pyridostigmine challenge	Patients with myasthenia gravis will improve in muscle strength and repetition for a short period of time following ingestion of this cholinesterase inhibitor

Diagnosis

Vertebral canal tumour

An insidious onset of neurological symptoms and more importantly cauda equina symptoms requires malignancy to be ruled out.

The gold standard investigation to confirm a vertebral canal tumour is an MRI spine..

Management

Medical

- Control modifiable risk factors: weight loss, regular exercise, smoking cessation
- Analgesia as required
- IV dexamethasone: anti-inflammatory and analgesia
- Manage any deformities associated with limb weakness or peripheral neuropathy:
  - Knee-ankle-foot orthosis (KAFO) for those with proximal weakness (e.g. trouble with knee extension and ankle dorsiflexion)
  - Ankle-foot orthosis (AFO) for those with foot drop/distal weakness
  - Physiotherapy
  - Pain relief or muscle relaxants for muscle spasms or contractures, e.g. baclofen, diazepam
  - Orthopaedic shoes
- Radiochemotherapy: some cancers can be reduced in size; it is best to discuss with neurosurgery specialists first, then the oncology team
  - Neoadjuvant, adjuvant therapy

Surgical

- Surgical treatment for vertebral metastasis is largely palliative (e.g. in radioresistant tumours such as sarcomas, lung, renal cell and colon cancers)
- Decompressive laminectomy is one such surgery that can be used for these patients who have intractable pain, have failed radiotherapy or have an unstable spine
- Biopsy: for tissue molecular and genetic diagnosis

Other differential diagnoses

- Compartment syndrome
- Vertebral disc bulge or herniation
- Cauda equina
- Myotonic dystrophy (Steinert's disease)
- Myasthenia gravis
- DMD
- Myositis

Station 44 **Lymphadenopathy**

A 60-year-old woman presents to the emergency department, referred by her GP for a CT scan showing diffuse lymphadenopathy.

Tasks

1 Take a history
2 Perform a targeted examination

3 Describe appropriate investigations
4 Formulate a management plan

Differential diagnoses (VIITAMINC)

Vascular:
- Kawasaki disease

Infective:
- Epstein–Barr virus (EBV)
- Streptococcal pharyngitis
- Tuberculosis
- Cytomegalovirus (CMV)
- Sexually-transmitted infection: HIV, gonococcal, syphilis, herpes simplex virus or *Chlamydia trachomatis*
- Toxoplasmosis (contact with cat faeces)
- Travel related: typhus, trypanosomiasis, leishmaniasis, typhoid

Inflammatory:
- Chronic granulomatous disease
- Localised – in response to a local skin infection

Traumatic:
- Cat scratch disease: cervical or axillary adenopathy

Autoimmune:
- Autoimmune lymphoproliferative syndrome
- Systemic lupus erythematosus (SLE)
- Sarcoidosis

Metabolic

Iatrogenic:
- Secondary to silicone breast implants: axillary lymphadenopathy
- Antihypertensives: atenolol, captopril, hydralazine
- Antimalarial medication
- Antibiotics: cephalosporins, penicillins, sulphonamides
- Anti-epileptics: carbamazepine, phenytoin

Neoplastic:
- Lymphoma
- Kaposi's sarcoma
- Leukaemia (the most common form of cancer in children)
- Lymphatic metastasis from any cancer

Congenital / **C**hromosomal:
- Common variable immunodeficiency
- Haemophagocytic syndrome

Other:
- Silicosis, asbestosis
- Lead, tyre or coal manufacturing
- Paint fumes

Before starting

Establish rapport:
▨ Introduce yourself
▨ Obtain consent from the patient to take a history from them and examine them
▨ Expose the patient: when physical examination is required

Confirm patient details:
▨ Name   *Fiona Richards*
▨ Age   *60 years*
▨ Occupation   *Translator*

History

History of presenting complaint (SOCRATES)

▨ **S**ite: *initially noted a lump above collar bone on the right 3 months ago, then noticed another on left neck yesterday*
▨ **O**nset: *first noticed 3 months ago*
▨ **C**haracter: *hard lump, doesn't seem to move; not painful to touch*
▨ **R**adiation: *no*
▨ **A**ssociated features: *has noticed increased sweating at night despite cooler weather; maybe some loss of weight but is always trying to lose some weight; there are also a lot of bruises on arms and legs, which is normal, but has just noticed some on back as well*
▨ **T**ime course: *no overseas travel recently*
▨ **E**xacerbating/relieving factors: *no*
▨ **S**everity: *the lumps seemed to have grown in size quite dramatically lately; can feel three lumps, the one above the collarbone may be 2cm in size, though the others are smaller*

Take a focused history

▨ Sick contacts: *no*
▨ Contact with TB- or HIV-infected persons: *no*
▨ Sexual history: *regular with husband of 35 years*
▨ Menstrual history: *underwent menopause at age 49 years*
▨ Lower urinary tract obstructive symptoms: *no*

Past medical history and family history

▨ *Childhood asthma*
▨ *Mother had breast cancer at 70 years, father had type 2 diabetes mellitus*

Drug history and allergies

▨ *Ventolin PRN*
▨ *NKDA*

Social history

▨ Smoking history: *non-smoker*
▨ Alcohol and drugs history: *social drinker, nil illicit drugs*

Examination

General inspection (ABCD-V)

▨ **A**ppearance: *patient looks comfortable*
▨ **B**ody habitus: *overweight, BMI 26*
▨ **C**ognition: *patient is conscious and oriented*
▨ **D**evices/**D**rugs: *no*
▨ **V**itals: *BP 120/80mmHg, HR 65bpm and regular, RR 16 per minute; oxygen saturation at 100% on room air; afebrile*

Haematological examination

▨ Eyes:
  ● Scleral icterus: *no*
  ● Mucosal pallor including conjunctiva: *no*
  ● Fundal examination: papilloedema, toxoplasmosis, CMV or haemorrhages: *no*
▨ Mouth:
  ● Gum hypertrophy: *no*
  ● Mucosal/gum bleeding: *no*
  ● Glossitis: *no*
  ● Waldeyer's ring inflammation or hypertrophy: *no*
▨ Neck:
  ● Cervical and supraclavicular lymph nodes: *multiple palpable nodes on both the left and right cervical chain; all hard, immobile lumps approximately 0.3 × 0.4cm in size; palpable supraclavicular node on right, hard and immobile, approximately 2.5 × 3cm in size; no tenderness on palpation*
  ● Tracheal deviation: *no*

- Upper limbs and chest:
  - Inspection – *no to all*:
    - Pallor or reduced capillary refill
    - Rheumatoid arthritis
    - Muscle wasting
    - Bony deformity or masses
    - Gouty tophi
  - Palpation:
    - Lymph nodes at cubital fossa (trochlear nodes) and axilla: *possible lymphadenopathy palpable in right axilla*
  - Auscultation:
    - Breath and heart sounds: *dual heart sounds, no murmur; normal breath sounds bilaterally*
    - *Globally reduced breath sounds can be due to a chronic obstructive lung disease, that predisposes to lung cancers*
    - *Focally reduced breath sounds can be due to pneumonia or obstructive mass*
- Abdomen:
  - Inspection:

- Jaundice, bowel distension, caput medusae: *no*
  - Palpation:
    - Hepatomegaly and splenomegaly: *mild splenomegaly palpated*
    - Abdominal mass: *no*
  - Auscultation:
    - *Normal bowel sounds*
- Lower limbs:
  - Inspection:
    - Petechiae, bruising, haematoma or rashes: *no*
    - *Pallor from anaemia*
    - Peripheral ulcerations: *no*
    - Muscle wasting: *no*
    - Lymphadenitis, infection or open wound: *no*
  - Palpation:
    - Popliteal and inguinal lymph node enlargement: *no*
    - *Power, sensation and reflexes intact and normal bilaterally*

Investigations

BBMI-O: Bedside, **B**loods, **M**icrobiology, **I**maging and **O**ther

Investigation	Rationale
Bedside	
Bloods	
FBC	Blood dyscrasias and white cell differential
CRP	Acute inflammation
ESR	Chronic inflammatory diseases
Viral serology for CMV, EBV, HIV	Chronic viral illnesses
QuantiFERON Gold (for TB)	Tuberculosis
Microbiology	
Throat culture	Streptococcus pharyngitis or EBV
First pass urine	Chlamydia or gonorrhoea
US-guided fine needle aspirate or CT-guided biopsy of a suspicious lymph node (>10mm in diameter)	Inflammatory disease versus neoplasm or metastasis

Investigation	Rationale
▦ Lymph node biopsy	▦ Working diagnosis of lymphoma
▦ Laparoscopic lymph node biopsies	▦ If lymph nodes are difficult to reach via CT or US-guided biopsy
Imaging	
▦ CXR	▦ Hilar lymphadenopathy, mediastinal mass or infection
▦ CT chest / abdomen / pelvis	▦ Infection, effusions, lung nodules or metastases
▦ PET ± lymphoscintigraphy	▦ Cancer – aids staging and surgical planning
Other	

Diagnosis

Lymphoma

An older patient with B symptoms and enlarged lymph nodes (especially supraclavicular) must be investigated thoroughly for lymphoma.

Discussion

Lymphoma is malignancy of the lymphatic system: an uncontrolled, abnormal growth of lymphocytes.

Categories:
▦ Hodgkin's lymphoma (HL): presence of Reed–Sternberg cells
▦ Non-Hodgkin's lymphoma (NHL): 90% of all lymphoma cases

Management

Medical

▦ Chemoradiotherapy:
  • NHL: localised radiotherapy alone or combined chemoradiotherapy; if aggressive stage, chemotherapy is commenced immediately
  • HL: combination of chemotherapy and radiotherapy; radiotherapy alone for bulky / non-responsive sites

▦ Monoclonal antibody therapy (i.e. rituximab): specific treatment with targeted therapy to a certain antigen
▦ Stem cell transplant: autologous (more common) and allogeneic; allows the use of higher chemotherapy doses

Surgical

▦ Not mainstay treatment; commonly used as a diagnostic process
▦ Resection of lymphoma indications: primary pulmonary disease (especially bronchus-associated lymph tissue, BALT), splenic lymphoma, nodal marginal zone lymphoma
▦ Intercostal catheter to drain pleural effusions, a complication of NHL

Other differential diagnoses

▦ Metastatic breast cancer
▦ Lymphadenitis

Station 45 **Melaena**

A 75-year-old man presents to your practice with a 3-day history of melaena.

Tasks

1 Take a history
2 Perform a targeted examination
3 Describe appropriate investigations
4 Formulate a management plan

Differential diagnoses (VIITAMINC)

Vascular:
- Angiodysplasia of gastrointestinal (GI) tract
- Arteriovenous malformations
- Gastric antral vascular ectasia (GAVE – uncommon)
- Mallory–Weiss syndrome
- Oesophageal varices

Infective:
- Parasites (unusual cause of upper GI bleeding)
- Tuberculosis

Inflammatory:
- Peptic ulcer disease / gastrointestinal ulcer
- Cameron lesions
- Erosive or severe oesophagitis
- Erosive or severe gastritis / duodenitis

Trauma:
- Oesophageal or GI foreign body

Autoimmune:
- Crohn's disease

Metabolic:
- Haemorrhagic disease of the newborn
- Liver failure
- Portal venous gastropathy (secondary to liver failure)

Idiopathic / **I**atrogenic:
- Gastrointestinal polyps
- Bleeding after medical or surgical interventions such as:
  - Aorto-enteric fistulas
  - Tetracycline
  - Post-surgical anastomotic bleeding
  - Meckel's diverticulum

Neoplasia:
- Upper gastrointestinal cancer

Congenital:
- Congenital coagulopathy
- Hereditary haemorrhagic telangiectasia
- Peutz–Jeghers syndrome

Before starting

Establish rapport:
- Introduce yourself
- Obtain consent from the patient to take a history from them and examine them
- Expose the patient: when physical examination is required
- Explain to the patient that you will need to do a rectal examination and consider need for chaperone

Confirm patient details:

Name	*Andrew Woods*
Age	*75 years*
Occupation	*Retired publican*

History

History of presenting complaint (SOCRATES)

- **S**ite: *black faeces*
- **O**nset: *3 days ago*

Character: *eight large liquid, tar-like motions each day; very smelly, "my wife can't enter the bathroom afterwards for hours"*

Radiation: *no*

Associated features: *no pain, loss of weight, fevers or vomiting*

Time course: *occurs frequently, after meals especially*

Exacerbating / relieving factors: *no*

Severity: *today starting to feel short of breath and dizzy on standing, a lot more tired than usual*

Past medical history and family history

Osteoarthritis in both knees, type 2 diabetes (diet controlled)

Father had heart attack at 65 years

Drug history and allergies

Recently started on NSAIDs for knee pain, otherwise no other medications

NKDA

Social history

Smoking history: *25 pack-years*

Alcohol and drugs history: *social drinker, nil illicit drugs*

Examination

General inspection (ABCD-V)

Appearance: *patient looks comfortable*

Body habitus: *overweight, BMI 26*

Cognition: *patient is conscious and oriented*

Devices / **D**rugs: *no*

Vitals: *BP 78/50mmHg, HR 122bpm and regular, RR 20 per minute; oxygen saturation at 94% on room air; afebrile*

Cardiovascular examination

Inspection:
  - Position the patient with their head and chest at 45 degrees
  - Surgical scars or abnormalities: *no*

Palpation:
  - Feel for the patient's pulse while simultaneously feeling for peripheral warmth and capillary refill:
    ▸ *Capillary refill >2 seconds ± peripherally cold is an indication of hypovolaemia*
  - Apex beat: *palpable at mid-clavicular line 5th intercostal space*
  - Heave / thrills: *no*

Percussion:
  - Effusions, dullness to percuss the posterior chest: *no*

Auscultation:
  - Heart sounds: *dual, no murmurs*
  - Lungs: *breath sounds normal globally*

Gastrointestinal examination

Look for:
  - Conjunctival pallor (anaemia)
  - Scleral icterus (hepatic failure)
  - Jaundice
  - Cutaneous haemangiomas:
    ▸ Presence of >5 suggests the possibility of gastrointestinal haemangiomas
  - Skin and mucosal bleeding, petechiae and bruising (coagulopathy)
  - Mucocutaneous telangiectasia
  - Midline sternotomy scars or radial artery graft harvest
  - Abdominal scars or wounds from recent surgical intervention
  - Lower limbs for saphenous vein harvest for coronary artery bypass graft, peripheral oedema, missing limbs or toes secondary to vascular disease

Gastrointestinal:
  - Inspection:
    ▸ Surgical scars or abnormalities: *no*
    ▸ Signs of portal venous hypertension – ascites, caput medusae: *no*
  - Palpation:
    ▸ Feel the abdomen for hepatosplenomegaly: *no*

- ▷ Epigastric tenderness: *mild epigastric tenderness on palpation*
- ▷ Note if any masses are felt on your examination: *no*
- Percussion:
  - ▷ *Normal resonant abdomen*
- Auscultation:
  - ▷ Bowel sounds: *mildly hyperactive bowel sounds*

Per rectal (PR) examination MUST be performed

- ▓ *No external deformity, anal fissures or haemorrhoids*
- ▓ *Melaena on digital rectal exam*

Investigations

BBMI-O: Bedside, **B**loods, **M**icrobiology, **I**maging and **O**ther

Investigation	Rationale
Bedside	
Bloods	
▓ FBC	▓ Infection and anaemia
▓ U&Es and creatinine	▓ Kidney function as a marker for dehydration secondary to hypovolaemia from blood loss
▓ LFTs	▓ Hepatic failure
▓ Coagulation profile	▓ Coagulopathy
▓ Iron studies	▓ Iron deficiency
Microbiology	
▓ Faecal occult blood test	▓ Bleeding from the bowel
Imaging	
▓ Plain AXR	▓ Metallic foreign body and complications such as bowel perforation or bowel obstruction
▓ CT abdomen / pelvis ± angiography	▓ Gastrointestinal masses; CT angiography is useful if suspecting an angiodysplastic mass
▓ Radionucleotide imaging of abdomen	▓ Most sensitive radiographic test for GI bleeding that occurs intermittently, e.g. Meckel's diverticulum
▓ Magnetic resonance enteropathy	▓ Able to differentiate between inflammatory and fibrotic disease
Other	
▓ Colonoscopy ± biopsies	▓ Looking for areas of thickened bowel wall, inflamed bowel wall; positive biopsies would be indicative of malignancy

Diagnosis

Ulcerated peptic ulcer

In an elderly patient with acute GI bleeding associated with meals and recent NSAID use, peptic ulcer disease is the primary differential.

Management

First principles of management in a patient with any bleed, upper GI included, are the principles of advanced life support (ALS) – **A**irway, **B**reathing, **C**irculation, **D**isability and **E**xposure. Ensure the patient is adequately resuscitated before surgical intervention is considered. One or more of the medical management options may be needed first.

Medical

- Cease the offending medications: in this case NSAIDs
- Anti-emetics to prevent vomiting if coinciding with melaena
- Resuscitation with blood products and / or replacement of iron with infusion or oral supplementation if also iron-deficient
- Replace haemoglobin (Hb) if <80g/L (8g/dl) in someone with cardiac disease, or <70g/L (7g/dl) in an otherwise healthy person; this threshold may differ in various health care services; replenish Hb with packed red blood cells: one unit will bring the Hb up approximately 10g/L (1g/dl)
- Withhold anticoagulants (when applicable)
- Reverse coagulopathy if able – discuss with Haematology
- Commence a proton pump inhibitor – pantoprazole, esomeprazole, etc.
- Radiologic angiography ± embolisation:
  - Requires active blood loss of 0.5–1.0ml/min and is reserved in patients that have haemodynamic instability and therefore are unable to undergo endoscopy

Surgical

- In patients presenting with unexplained GI bleeding more than one teaspoon of blood loss, a nasogastric tube is helpful to confirm the bleed is ongoing
- Endoscopy:
  - First-line treatment for an actively bleeding upper GI lesion which can be treated with an injection of adrenaline or sclerosant, haemoclip placement and band ligation for varices, and thermal cauterisation for ulcerations or gastritis
  - Helpful in identifying an aortoenteric fistula
- Colonoscopy:
  - If bleeding is not identified with an endoscopy, a colonoscopy may be useful to identify the source
- Wireless capsule endoscopy:
  - Useful if bleeding is intermittent or unable to be identified despite endoscopy and colonoscopy; this is called a 'Pillcam', which is an ingested camera slightly larger than a standard pharmaceutical tablet, and takes photos as it travels through the gastrointestinal system
- Surgical repair:
  - Exploratory laparotomy should be considered in patients with suspected aortoenteric fistula with severe ongoing bleeding:
    - Approach involves repair of an aortic aneurysm and fistula

Other differential diagnoses

- Oesophageal variceal bleeding
- Crohn's disease

Station 46 **Mouth ulcer**

A 45-year-old man presents to the GP complaining of a mouth ulcer.

Tasks

1   Take a history
2   Perform a targeted examination

3   Describe appropriate investigations
4   Formulate a management plan

Differential diagnoses (VIITAMINC)

Vascular:
- Vasculitic disorders:
  - Behçet's disease – ulcerations in the mouth and on genitals
  - Granulomatosis with polyangiitis (90% of patients have oral ulcerations)
  - Kawasaki disease

Infective:
- Herpetic (including stomatitis and gingivostomatitis)
- Tonsillitis
- Coxsackie virus (hand, foot and mouth disease)
- Herpangina
- Bacterial and parasitic causes:
  - Gonorrhoea
  - Syphilis
  - *Helicobacter pylori*
  - Leishmaniasis

Inflammatory:
- Inflammatory bowel disease
- Coeliac disease
- Rheumatoid diseases (e.g. Behçet's)

Trauma:
- From ill-fitting dentures or sharp, broken teeth or stomatitis

Autoimmune:

- Stevens–Johnson syndrome – oral involvement in >90% of patients
- Lichen planus
- Pemphigus vulgaris
- Paraneoplastic pemphigus (PNP)
- Desquamative gingivitis
- Benign mucous membrane pemphigoid
- Subacute cutaneous lupus erythematosus (SCLE)

Metabolic:
- Iron-deficiency anaemia
- Folate deficiency

Iatrogenic:
- Recurrent aphthous ulcers (RAS)
- Major aphthous ulcers
- Medications:
  - Methotrexate, foscarnet, interferon, nicorandil, chemotherapy drugs

Neoplasia:
- Oral squamous cell carcinoma (SCC)
- Pre-neoplastic: leukoplakia
- Oral proliferative verrucous leukoplakia
- Rare pre-neoplastic lesion: erythroplakia
- Kaposi's sarcoma

Congenital:
- As per autoimmune causes

Before starting

Establish rapport:
- Introduce yourself
- Obtain consent from the patient to take a history from them and examine them
- Expose the patient: when physical examination is required

Confirm patient details:
- Name   *David Donaldson*
- Age   *45 years*
- Occupation   *Accountant*

History

History of presenting complaint (SOCRATES)

- **S**ite: *self-explanatory*
- **O**nset: *started 3 days ago, progressively worsening*
- **C**haracter: *multiple ulcers in the cheeks and roof of the mouth, some coming up on lips now as well; all are relatively small in size, though are associated with blisters*
- **R**adiation: *nil*
- **A**ssociated features: *painful constantly, associated with a burning sensation; no blood*
- **T**ime course: *3 days now; has had similar things occur in the past a couple of times in the last year, though not as bad*
- **E**xacerbating / relieving factors: *worse on eating / drinking*
- **S**everity: *the pain has affected the ability to eat and drink*

Past medical history and family history

- *Nil significant past medical history*
- *Father had chronic obstructive pulmonary disease (COPD)*

Drug history and allergies

- *Nil*
- *NKDA*

Social history

- Smoking history: *15 pack-years*
- Alcohol and drugs history: *4 beers per day, nil illicit drugs*
- *Recently divorced, currently undertaking legal battles for custody of the children; has had multiple new sexual partners in the last few months*

Examination

General inspection (ABCD-V)

- **A**ppearance: *patient looks comfortable*
- **B**ody habitus: *normal, BMI 23*
- **C**ognition: *patient is conscious and oriented*
- **D**evices / **D**rugs: *nil*
- **V**itals: *BP 118/75mmHg, HR 68bpm and regular; afebrile*

Mouth examination

- Inspection: *multiple pin-head sized vesicles surrounding the left angle of the mouth, and on the frenulum; gingivitis noted throughout the whole mouth*
- Palpation: *vesicles are tender to touch*

Investigations

BBMI-O: Bedside, **B**loods, **M**icrobiology, **I**maging and **O**ther

Investigation	Rationale
Bedside	
Bloods	
▣ FBC + WCC with differential	▣ Infection, anaemia, neutropenia
▣ B$_{12}$, folate, iron studies	▣ Deficiency
▣ CRP	▣ Acute marker of inflammation
▣ Serum antiendomysium Ab ± transglutaminase assay	▣ Positive result in coeliac disease
▣ Calcium level	▣ A poor prognostic factor primarily found in persons with advanced disease
▣ Serum alpha-antitrypsin, alpha-antiglycoprotein levels	▣ Head and neck cancer may increase levels of these proteins in the blood
Microbiology	
Imaging	
▣ Laryngoscopy	▣ Extent of cancer and any further lesions, also to document vocal cord function prior to any oropharyngeal surgery
▣ CT and MRI head and neck	▣ Aid surgical planning for removal and to identify invasion into surrounding structures or metastasis
▣ CT chest/abdomen/pelvis + PET (18-FDG positive electron tomography)	▣ Staging scans for operative and adjunct medical management
Other	
▣ Swab/scraping MCS	▣ Looking for HSV type 1
▣ Biopsy of the lesion if suspecting inflammatory or neoplastic cause	▣ Differentiate between inflammatory disease and neoplasms such as Behçet's versus SCC
▣ US-guided lymph node FNA for cytology	▣ If suspecting a lymph node metastasis or concurrent lymphadenopathy

Diagnosis

Herpetic gingivostomatitis (HSV type 1)

A patient with past history of a similar presentation and vesicles around the mouth is suggestive of HSV-1.

The gold standard investigation for HSV-1 is lesion swab MCS ± polymerase chain reaction.

Discussion

- Combination of gingivitis (inflammation of the gums) and stomatitis (inflammation of the lips/mouth)
- Often the initial presentation during the primary HSV infection, which is the most common viral infection of the mouth
- Generally, lesions heal spontaneously within 7–14 days in healthy individuals

Looking at...	Oral ulcer type		
	Cancerous	Aphthous	Herpetic gingivostomatitis
Time course	Present for >3 weeks. Patient may have noticed erythroplakia or leukoplakia prior to the ulcer formation	No prodrome. <6 ulcers that self-resolve then recur within 1–4 months	If left untreated, last 14+ days; may recur multiple times a year
Age group	40+ years old	Any (usually children to early adults)	Acute form: children 6 months to 6 years (has features of systemic illness). Chronic, recurrent form: most often affects adults, do not experience systemic illness
Precipitating causes	Smoking, alcohol excess, betel nut use, HPV (hepatitis C also increases risk)	Emotional stress, local trauma, food allergies, autoimmune disease flare	Sunlight, fever, immunosuppression, emotional stress
Associated features	Weight loss, malaise, fevers, loss of appetite, difficulty swallowing due to mass, change in voice or hoarseness, bleeding or pain in the mouth, locoregional lymphadenopathy	Painful, the patient may avoid salty, hot or spicy foods	Severe mouth pain ± fever, malaise, loss of appetite
Location	Tongue and the floor of mouth most common	Non-keratinised mucosa + tongue	Around the lips or buccal mucosa

Looking at...	Oral ulcer type		
	Cancerous	Aphthous	Herpetic gingivostomatitis
Ulcer bed	Irregular borders, with erosion or exophytic mass; in the advanced stage, it may present as an ulcer with a large raised border	Small, well defined, round ulcer with shallow yellow or grey base	Vesicles that form from multiple pin-head sized ulcers <5mm in diameter; these then coalesce and leave large, ragged ulcers
Surrounding tissue	May be tethered or indurated; may have erythroplakia or leukoplakia	May have a halo of erythema but no induration or tethering	Lesions usually grouped in small clusters

Management

Lifestyle

- Good oral hygiene
- Brush teeth with a small-headed, soft toothbrush
- Avoid eating hard or sharp foods (e.g. crisps, toast)
- Adequate fluid intake
- If a patient relates oral ulcers to her menstrual cycle, the use of an oral contraceptive may aid to suppress ovulation
- Minimise intimate contact when lesions are active to reduce the viral spread

Medical

- Goals of treatment – relief of pain and reduction of ulcer duration:
  - If recurrent aphthous ulcerations, mainstays of treatment are topical corticosteroids, e.g. triamcinolone, hydrocortisone, betamethasone mouth rinse; NB: betamethasone, fluocinonide, fluticasone and clobetasol are more potent steroids and carry the possibility of some adrenocortical suppression and predisposition to candidiasis
  - Chlorhexidine gluconate mouth rinses reduce the severity and pain of ulceration, but do not affect frequency
  - Topical anti-inflammatory immuno-modulator paste reduces healing time, accelerates pain resolution, and prevents recurrences – recommended only if there is only one lesion
- Replace deficient vitamins and minerals (B_{12}, folate, iron)
- Antivirals: aciclovir (Zovirax):
  - Inhibits the activity of HSV-1 and HSV-2
  - Prescribed for immunocompromised and immunocompetent patients

Surgical

- Debridement: gentle removal of the infected tissue (especially in gangrenous cases)

Other differential diagnoses

- Kawasaki disease
- Neoplastic: oral squamous cell carcinoma

Station 47 **Muscle weakness**

An 80-year-old woman presents to the GP with a difficulty in lifting her left leg.

Tasks

1 Take a history

2 Perform a targeted examination

3 Describe appropriate investigations

4 Formulate a management plan

Differential diagnoses (VIITAMINC) *(*1–2 muscles affected only)*

Vascular:
- Polyarteritis nodosa
- Isolated peripheral nervous system vasculitis
- Mononeuritis multiplex

Infective:
- Herpes simplex, Epstein–Barr and herpes zoster viruses

Inflammatory:
- Myositis

Trauma:
- Muscle or tendon separation from the insertion point
- Brachial plexus syndrome*
- Axillary nerve injury*
- Suprascapular neuropathy*
- Compressive: carpal tunnel syndrome, pronator teres syndrome, ulnar neuropathy
- Radial neuropathy*
- Sciatic neuropathy
- Spinal accessory neuropathy*
- Deep fibular nerve injury*

Autoimmune:
- Multiple sclerosis
- Hypo- and hyperthyroidism
- Myositis

Metabolic:
- Hypokalaemia
- B$_{12}$ deficiency
- Lead and mercury poisoning
- Glucocorticoid excess (i.e. Cushing's syndrome)
- Acid maltase deficiency

Idiopathic / **I**atrogenic:
- Polymyalgia rheumatica
- Guillain–Barré syndrome
- Spinal canal stenosis
- Idiopathic myopathy
- Drug-induced myopathy: amiodarone, chloroquine, heroin, lithium, misoprostol, nitrofurantoin, vincristine, statins
- Amyotrophic lateral sclerosis

Neoplasia:
- Sarcoma with consequent nerve compression
- Central nervous system tumour
- Paraneoplastic phenomena

Congenital:
- Charcot–Marie–Tooth disease
- Congenital muscular dystrophy
- Juvenile amyotrophic lateral sclerosis

Before starting

Establish rapport:
- Introduce yourself
- Obtain consent from the patient to take a history and examine the patient

- Expose the patient: when physical examination is required

Confirm patient details:
- Name — *Thérèse Delafoy*
- Age — *80 years*
- Occupation — *Retired seamstress*

History

History of presenting complaint (SOCRATES)

▨ **S**ite: *left leg, entire leg feels weak*
▨ **O**nset:
  ● *Initially noticed a month ago, though sudden progression to loss of strength today*
  ● Precipitating traumatic event: *no*
▨ **C**haracter:
  ● Constant: *yes*
  ● Most difficult movement to do: *bend / stretch the leg*
▨ **R**adiation: *no*
▨ **A**ssociated features:
  ● Pop or crack at the time of injury: *no*
  ● Fevers, rigors, chills: *no*
  ● 'B symptoms': *possible weight loss over the last couple of months, feeling more and more fatigued lately but attributed that to age*
  ● Unable to descend stairs or a feeling of their knee 'giving way' when walking: *no*
  ● Swelling, pain or erythema in the affected region: *no*
  ● Bruising: *no*
  ● Sensory changes: *yes, the leg also feels heavier and numb*
  ● Symptoms worsen with heat or exercise: *no*
▨ **T**ime course: *as above*
▨ **E**xacerbating / relieving factors: *none*
▨ **S**everity: *unable to perform activities of daily life as cannot walk properly*
  ● Pain: *no pain in the leg, though has noticed a headache which won't leave over the last month that seems to be worsening*

Past medical history and family history

▨ *Nil significant past medical history*
▨ *No family history*

Drug history and allergies

▨ *Currently just on medications for hypertension – unable to remember name*

Social history

▨ Smoking history: *non-smoker*
▨ Alcohol and drugs history: *non-drinker, nil illicit drugs*

▨ *Lives at home with husband; children help out with the house maintenance*

Examination

General inspection (ABCD-V)

▨ **A**ppearance: *patient looks comfortable*
▨ **B**ody habitus: *normal, BMI 22*
▨ **C**ognition: *patient is conscious and oriented*
▨ **D**evices / **D**rugs: *no*
▨ **V**itals: *BP 140/98mmHg, HR 98bpm and regular, RR 18 per minute; oxygen saturation at 99% on room air; afebrile*

Lower limb examination

▨ Inspection:
  ● Rashes: *no*
  ● Muscle wasting: *yes, the left thigh is smaller than the right*
  ● Obvious deformity: *no*
  ● Oedema or localised swelling related to a fracture or joint disruption: *no*
  ● Overlying bruising on the affected limb / muscle: *no*
▨ Palpation:
  ● Crepitus: *no*
  ● Clear steps or deformities under the skin: *no*
  ● Temperature between both limbs affected and compare them: *normal bilaterally*
  ● Capillary refill in the affected limb: *<2 seconds*
  ● Masses: *no*
  ● Tenderness over the origin and insertion points of the muscles affected: *no*
  ● *Strong arterial pulses bilaterally*
▨ Move:
  ● Tone: *normal*
  ● Power: *entire left leg 4/5, right leg 5/5 globally*
  ● Proximal myopathy: *difficulty standing from sitting as unbalanced from the lack of strength in left leg*

Neurological examination

▨ Sensation: *reduced sensation throughout the left leg, right leg normal*
▨ Reflexes: *slight hyper-reflexia on the left knee, otherwise normal*
▨ Proprioception: *normal*

Investigations

BBMI-O: Bedside, **B**loods, **M**icrobiology, **I**maging and **O**ther

Investigation	Rationale
Bedside	
Bloods	
▦ FBC	▦ Infection and anaemia
▦ CRP	▦ Acute marker of inflammation
▦ U&Es and creatinine	▦ Looking at renal function and electrolytes
▦ Anti-acetylcholinesterase receptor Abs	▦ Myasthenia gravis
▦ Anti-endomysium and anti-AGA Abs	▦ Myositis
▦ TFTs	▦ Thyroid disease
▦ Chromosomal analysis	▦ Genetic disorder for muscular dystrophy
Microbiology	
Imaging	
▦ X-ray of affected limb (anterior-posterior view, lateral and oblique views)	▦ Looking for a fracture, dislocation or joint separation
▦ MRI of affected region	▦ An underlying compressive mass, or tear in a ligament, tendon or muscle belly; also aids in surgical planning
▦ MRI / CT brain	▦ Looking for cranial pathology
Other	
▦ Muscle or lesion biopsy	▦ Myositis or to characterise a mass
▦ 24-hour urine heavy metal titres – if a history of lead or mercury exposure	▦ Heavy metal toxicity
▦ EMG and nerve conduction studies	▦ Can aid differentiation of intrinsic neuropathy, myasthenia gravis or myopathy

Diagnosis

Intracranial tumour

An elderly patient with unintentional loss of weight, fatigue, headache and upper motor symptoms unilaterally (muscle wasting, weakness, hyperreflexia) is very suspicious for intracranial malignancy.

The gold standard investigation to confirm an intracranial tumour is an MRI brain.

Management

Medical

- Physiotherapy input:
  - Knee-ankle-foot orthosis (KAFO) for those with proximal weakness (i.e. trouble with knee extension and ankle dorsiflexion)
  - Ankle-foot orthosis (AFO) for those with foot drop / distal weakness
- Analgesia as required
- Chemotherapy: neoadjuvant and adjuvant therapy in combination with radiotherapy
- Radiotherapy: commonly in combination with chemotherapy initially and then continued alone; stereotactic radiosurgery is precise form of radiation that utilises small direct beams, utilised in cases where tumours are in close proximity to critical structures

Surgical

- Neurosurgical input for tumour resection or debulking

Other differential diagnoses

- Fracture (femur, tibia / fibula)
- Muscular or tendon sprain / strain

Station 48 **Nail changes**

An 18-year-old man presents to your GP practice with the complaint of an acute isolated nail change.

Tasks

1 Take a history
2 Perform a targeted examination
3 Name at least three potential differential diagnoses
4 Describe appropriate investigations
5 Formulate a management plan

Differential diagnoses

Nail colour:
- Leukonychia
- Yellow nail syndrome

Nail bed:
- Paronychia
- Melanoma striata
- Cancers
  - Warty dyskeratoma
  - Glomus tumour: rare benign tumour, blue lesion under the nail plate
  - Squamous cell carcinoma (SCC) *in situ*
  - Amelanotic melanoma
  - Malignant melanoma
  - Nail fibroma
- Mucous cysts

Nail plate:
- Clubbing
- Trachyonychia
- Splinter haemorrhages
- Nail plate disruption ('onycholysis')
- Onychomycosis (fungal nail infection)
- Onychogryphosis (goat horn nail)
- Subungual hyperkeratosis
- Nail plate irregularity with ridging
- Pitting

Nail fold:
- Human papillomavirus
- Verruca wart
- Malignant melanoma

Before starting

Establish rapport:
- Introduce yourself
- Obtain consent to take a history and examine the patient
- Expose the patient when physical examination is required

Confirm patient details:
- Name   *Mitchell Chapman*
- Age   *18 years*
- Occupation   *Student*

History

History of presenting complaint (SOCRATES)

- **S**ite: *big toe on left foot*
- **O**nset: *changes first noted 1 month ago, has progressively worsened since then; first episode; no associated trauma / recent illness or change in diet; prior to this, the foot was quite red and itchy for a week*
- **C**haracter: *the nail appears yellow / cloudier and is thicker than the other nails, with part of the top broken off; the surrounding skin on the toe looks scaly*

Radiation: *no*

Associated features: *no*

Time course: *as per onset*

Exacerbating / relieving: *no*

Severity: *it is just ugly to look at and my mother told me I needed to get it looked at*

Past medical history and family history

No relevant past medical history

No relevant family history

Drug history and allergies

No regular medications

NKDA

Social history

Smoking history: *no*

Alcohol and drugs history: *social drinker, no illicit drugs*

Examination

General inspection (ABCD-V)

Appearance: *patient looks well*

Body habitus: *normal, BMI 20*

Cognition: *conscious and oriented*

Devices / **D**rugs: *nil*

Vitals: *all vital signs within normal limits; afebrile*

Hand / foot

Nails:

- *Inspection reveals a yellow / discoloured left toenail, which is thickened; several pieces appear to be breaking off the nail*

- *Surrounding skin is not erythematous; however, appears scaly*

- *No pitting, clubbing, leukonychia, koilonychia, Beau's lines, Mees' bands, Lindsay's nails or Terry's nails on examination*

Inspection of skin

Bleeding, ulceration, telangiectasia, lesions: *no*

Alopecia (hair loss): *no*

Angular stomatitis: *no*

Investigations

BBMI-O: Bedside, **B**loods, **M**icrobiology, **I**maging and **O**ther

Investigation	Rationale
Bloods	
FBC	Infection and anaemia
CRP	Acute marker of inflammation
U&Es and creatinine	Renal disease
LFTs	Liver disease
Glucose level and HbA1c	Diabetes and its control
Iron studies, B_{12}	Causes of anaemia and nail plate ridging

Investigation	Rationale
Microbiology	
Biopsy of the lesion if suspecting an inflammatory or neoplastic cause	Differentiate between inflammatory disease and neoplasms
Nail pus swab for MCS (if paronychia)	To rule out MRSA infection
Nail clippings for mycology	Fungal infection
Imaging	
X-ray of affected limb and foot	Osteomyelitis or underlying fracture if investigating traumatic nail injury

Diagnosis

Fungal nail infection (onychomycosis)

Management

Lifestyle

- Control modifiable risk factors: feet hygiene (clean and dry), wearing breathable footwear, protecting feet in shared bathrooms, changing socks often

Medical

- Topical azole cream for immunocompetent patients
- Oral antifungal agents: e.g. daily terbinafine (first line) or 'pulse therapy' with oral itraconazole for 1 week each month for 3–4 months, fluconazole once weekly until nail is normal (first line in candida infections)
- Chemical nail avulsion: urea ointment

Surgical

- Biopsy of lesion (excisional biopsy)
  - May need to remove nail plate if lesion is within nail bed

Other differential diagnoses

- Paronychia
- Ingrown nail
- SCC *in situ*
- Malignant melanoma (subungual)

Station 49 **Neck lump**

A 75-year-old man presents to the GP with a left-sided neck lump.

Tasks

1 Take a history
2 Perform a targeted examination

3 Describe appropriate investigations
4 Formulate a management plan

Differential diagnoses (VIITAMINC)

Vascular:
- Haemangioma
- Pyogenic granuloma

Infective:
- Inflammatory reactive lymphadenopathy – cervical (most common in children)
- Epstein–Barr virus (EBV)
- Bacterial lymphadenopathy
- Peritonsillar abscess (quinsy)
- Retropharyngeal abscess
- Dental abscess with localised lymphadenopathy
- Epiglottitis

Inflammatory

Trauma:
- Haematoma from a recent injury

Autoimmune

Metabolic:
- Thyroid goitre

Iatrogenic

Neoplasia:
- Thyroid mass:

- Multinodular goitre
- Thyroid cancer
- Parathyroid adenoma
- Tongue base disorder (usually squamous cell carcinoma)
- Tonsillar cancer
- Schwannoma (superior cervical sympathetic chain or vagus nerve)
- Lipoma
- Epidermoid inclusion cysts
- Submandibular gland tumour
- Nasopharyngeal carcinoma
- Infantile fibrosarcoma
- Dermoid cyst

Congenital:
- Thyroglossal duct cyst
- Branchial cleft cyst
- Laryngocele – herniation of saccule of the larynx
- Ranula
- Teratoma
- Dermoid cyst
- Thymic cyst
- Infantile myofibromatosis

Other

Before starting

Establish rapport:
- Introduce yourself
- Obtain consent from the patient to take a history from them and examine them

- Expose the patient: when physical examination is required

Confirm patient details:
- Name   *Barry Sign*
- Age   *75 years*
- Occupation   *Retired, previous warehouse worker*

History

History of presenting complaint (SOCRATES)

- **S**ite: *left side of the neck, 2–3cm above the sternum*
- **O**nset: *noticed the lump first 8 months ago, may have got bigger in this time*
- **C**haracter: *mild pressure sensation*
- **R**adiation: *no*
- **A**ssociated features:
  - Shortness of breath (dyspnoea): *no*
  - Pharyngitis, rhinorrhoea, otalgia: *no*
  - Odynophagia: *no*
  - Dysphagia: *no*
  - Oral cavity or oropharyngeal ulcer: *no*
  - Nasal congestion or epistaxis ipsilateral to a neck mass: *no*
  - Hoarseness or voice change: *no*
  - 'B symptoms': *some unexplained weight loss*
  - Drooling: *no*
  - Tripoding, stridor: *no*
- **T**ime course: *8 months, progressive increase in size*
- **E**xacerbating / relieving factors: *no*
- **S**everity: *constant lump, no fluctuation*

Past medical history and family history

- *Gastro-oesophageal reflux disease, mild chronic obstructive pulmonary disease (COPD)*
- *Mother had something cut out of her thyroid, father had COPD*

Drug history and allergies

- Medications: *esomeprazole 20mg daily, Ventolin PRN*
- *NKDA*

Social history

- Smoking history: *30 pack-years*
- Alcohol and drugs history: *3–4 drinks per day, nil illicit drugs*

Examination

General inspection (ABCD-V)

- **A**ppearance: *patient looks comfortable*
- **B**ody habitus: *obese, BMI 30*
- **C**ognition: *patient is conscious and oriented*
- **D**evices / **D**rugs: *no*
- **V**itals: *BP 140/98mmHg. HR is 98bpm and regular, RR 18 per minute; oxygen saturation at 99% on room air; afebrile*

Head and neck examination

- Inspection:
  - External head and neck:
    - *Patient looks well*
    - Obvious abnormalities of the face or neck: *no*
    - Location of mass: *3cm above jugular angle on the left upper thyroid lobe, no obvious goitre*
    - Ulceration, tethering or colour change of overlying skin: *no*
    - Skin lesions on the scalp, face or neck: *a couple of freckles and seborrhoeic keratoses*
  - Oropharynx:
    - Petechiae overlying mucosa: *no*
    - Active bleeding: *no*
    - Mass with overlying ulceration, tethering, pus or petechiae: *no*
    - Uvula displacement: *uvula is midline*
    - Vesicular formations overlying the pharynx: *no*
    - Oral candidiasis: *no*
    - Exudative erythematous pharyngitis with palatal petechiae: *no*
- Palpation:
  - Mass: *2 × 1cm nodule in the left upper lobe of the thyroid, no other palpable masses*
  - Texture: *firm and tethered nodule*
  - Tenderness: *non-tender on palpation*
  - Lymph nodes: *no palpable lymphadenopathy*
- Percussion:
  - Neck: *no retrosternal expansion noted*
  - Lungs: *no dullness on percussion*
- Auscultate:
  - Thyroid bruits: *no*
  - Lungs: *normal vesicular sounds bilaterally*

Cranial nerve examination

Normal

Investigations

BBMI-O: Bedside, **B**loods, **M**icrobiology, **I**maging and **O**ther

Investigation	Rationale
Bedside	
Bloods	
FBC	Infection, anaemia, pancytopenia
CRP	Acute marker of inflammation
Glucose level and HbA1c	Diabetes and its control
LFTs	Coagulopathy or if deranged, may be due to cancer metastases
LDH	Level of LDH to aid tumour staging
Microbiology	
Imaging	
CXR – lateral neck, AP	Retropharyngeal infection
CT neck with oral and IV contrast, MRI neck	Tumour mass characterisation through MRI and CT
Other	
FNA or core biopsy of the mass	Characterisation of mass
Laryngoscopy	If mass extends into or arises from the oropharynx; also to evaluate the function of vocal cords

Diagnosis

Thyroid cancer

A firm neck lump with insidious onset associated with unintentional weight loss in an elderly patient is very concerning for malignancy.

The gold standard investigation to confirm thyroid cancer is biopsy (FNA or core).

Discussion

Types of thyroid cancer:
- Papillary: most common, slow growing
- Follicular: slow growing, highly treatable
- Medullary: poorly differentiated
- Anaplastic: rare, aggressive type of poorly differentiated cancer

Management

Medical

- Chemotherapy ± radiotherapy: neoadjuvant and adjuvant
- Radioiodine: suitable for papillary or follicular thyroid cancer, as these tumours absorb the iodine; commenced 4–5 weeks post surgery
- Thyroxine: if total thyroidectomy to replace T_4

Surgical

- Hemi- or total thyroidectomy with preservation of thyroid glands where possible

Other differential diagnoses

- Haemangioma
- Retropharyngeal infection
- Metastatic skin cancer (squamous cell, basal cell, melanoma)
- Epiglottitis
- Quinsy

Station 50 **Odynophagia**

A 65-year-old man presents to the GP with increasing pain on swallowing food.

Tasks

1 Take a history
2 Perform a targeted examination

3 Describe appropriate investigations
4 Formulate a management plan

Differential diagnoses (VIITAMINC)

Vascular:
- Haemangioma

Infective:
- Oropharyngeal candidiasis
- Tonsillitis
- Peritonsillar abscess
- Epiglottitis
- Streptococcal pharyngitis
- Retropharyngeal abscess
- Bacterial tracheitis
- Uvulitis
- Viral pharyngitis

Inflammatory:
- Oesophagitis
- Gastro-oesophageal reflux disease (GORD)
- Oesophageal strictures

Trauma:
- Caustic or thermal burns to the posterior pharynx
- Foreign body

- Oesophageal or pharyngeal ulceration secondary to radiation for cancer
- Oesophageal perforation

Autoimmune

Metabolic

Iatrogenic:
- Recent placement of an endotracheal tube or laryngeal mask airway

Neoplastic:
- Malignancy of tongue base, pharynx or oesophagus

Congenital

Other:
- Achalasia
- Oesophageal dysmotility disorder

Before starting

Establish rapport:
- Introduce yourself
- Obtain consent to take a history and examine the patient
- Expose the patient: when physical examination is required

Confirm patient details:
- Name   *Alexander Price*
- Age   *65 years*
- Occupation   *Insurance salesman*

History

History of presenting complaint (SOCRATES)

- **S**ite: *in the central chest, sometimes coming up into the throat*
- **O**nset: *always after meals*
- **C**haracter: *burning type sensation, especially with spicy and acidic foods; no trouble swallowing or sensation of sticking*

- **R**adiation: *back of the throat; when this happens it is associated with an acidic taste and the feeling of wanting to vomit*
- **A**ssociated features:
  - Viral symptoms: *no, though has a dry cough which has been worsening*
  - 'B symptoms': *no*
  - Bruising easily, bleeding, or petechiae: *no*
  - Loss of appetite: *no*
  - Shortness of breath: *no*
  - Voice change: *no*
  - Food regurgitation: *no*
  - Aspiration, the feeling of choking or sticking: *no*
  - Chest pain, neck pain or dyspnoea: *no*
- **T**ime course: *over the last few months, initially sporadic every few days but now after every meal, even snacks*
- **E**xacerbating / relieving factors: *worse at night, especially on lying down; seems to be worse after spicy food and alcohol*
- **S**everity: *7/10 when present*

Past medical history and family history

- *Asthma, hypertension and type 2 diabetes*
- *Family history of 'reflux'*

Drug history and allergies

- *Enalapril, metformin, gliclazide, salbutamol MDI*
- *Allergic to amoxicillin: rash*

Social history

- Smoking history: *50 pack-years*

- Alcohol and drugs history: *5–8 beers/day, more on weekends, nil illicit drugs*
- *Lives at home alone*

Examination

General inspection (ABCD-V)

- **A**ppearance: *patient looks comfortable*
- **B**ody habitus: *obese, BMI 30*
- **C**ognition: *patient is conscious and oriented*
- **D**evices / **D**rugs: *no*
- **V**itals: *all within normal limits*

Oropharyngeal examination

- General inspection
  - Angular cheilitis: *no*
  - Angioedema: *no*
  - Herpes simplex ulcerations: *no*
  - Oral candidiasis (adherent white plaques over mucosa): *no*
  - Glossitis (inflammation of the tongue): *no*
  - Asymmetry of the soft palate (involvement of cranial nerves IX or X): *no*
  - Posterior pharynx: *normal*
- Palpation: *no palpable lymphadenopathy*

Respiratory

- Inspection: *patient looks slightly out of breath*
- Palpation: *normal*
- Percussion: *normal resonance*
- Auscultation: *mild-to-moderate globalised expiratory wheeze*

Investigations

BBMI-O: Bedside, **B**loods, **M**icrobiology, **I**maging and **O**ther

Investigation	Rationale
Bedside	
Bloods	
FBC	Infection and anaemia
CRP	Acute marker of inflammation
U&Es, creatinine, CMP	Electrolyte imbalances (caused by malnutrition)
Glucose level and HbA1c	Diabetes and its control (increased risk of infections)

Investigation	Rationale
Microbiology	
Biopsy of a lesion	Looking for malignancy
Blood cultures	Systemic infection
Group A streptococcus throat culture swab	Streptococcal pharyngitis
Viral throat swab	Viral cause of pharyngitis
Imaging	
CT	Obstructive mass in oesophagus or pharynx
MRI	Distinguishing between pharyngeal muscles from mucosa and lymph nodes (if a mass is found on CT)
PET	Metastatic cancer
Endoscopy and biopsy	Oesophageal mass or gastro-oesophageal reflux
Other	
Biopsy of a lesion	Differentiate between inflammatory disease and neoplasms
Flexible fibreoptic endoscopy	Laryngeal mass and to assess vocal cord function
Oesophageal manometry	Achalasia
Barium swallow	Looking for oesophagitis and causes of dysphagia
Urea breath test	Looking to diagnose *Helicobacter pylori*
CLO test (rapid urease test)	Looking to diagnose *H. pylori*; performed at time of endoscopy (gastroscopy) via biopsy

Diagnosis

Gastro-oesophageal reflux disease (GORD)

A burning pain following foods, exacerbated by spicy / acidic foods, and lying down, is typical of GORD.

Management

Medical

- Control modifiable risk factors:
  - Diabetes control, weight reduction, reduced meal sizes
  - Cease smoking, reduce or cease alcohol intake
- Ensure a period of time is taken between eating meals and lying down; raise the head of the bed
- Antacid: PRN therapy, liquid form is more effective than oral
- Proton pump inhibitor: esomeprazole, first-line therapy; trial for approximately 4–8 weeks in severe cases

- H$_2$ antagonist: ranitidine, as a nocturnal adjuvant
- Oesophageal dysmotility: calcium channel blockers as primary treatment

Surgical

- Endoscopic procedures
  - Resection of nodular areas in Barrett's oesophagus
  - Laparoscopic Nissen fundoplication: in patients with a symptomatic hiatus hernia who have failed medical management or severe GORD that has failed medical management

- Oesophageal dysmotility disorder that has failed conservative management:
  - Botulinum toxin injection to the oesophagus
  - Per-oral distal oesophageal sphincter myotomy

Other differential diagnoses

- Oesophageal candidiasis
- Oesophageal neoplasia
- Tonsillitis

Station 51 **Oliguria**

A 67-year-old man, day-3 postoperative surgical patient, is reported by nursing staff to have reduced urine output.

Tasks

1 Take a history
2 Perform a targeted examination

3 Describe appropriate investigations
4 Formulate a management plan

Differential diagnoses

Pre-renal causes:

- Hypovolaemia:
  - Inadequate fluid intake
  - Fluid loss:
    - Haemorrhage, via burns, hyperthermia, nephrotic syndrome
    - Gastrointestinal fluid loss: vomiting, diarrhoea, nasogastric suctioning
    - Fluid loss via kidneys: diuretics, glycosuria
  - Third-spacing of fluid: pancreatitis, bowel obstruction
- Cardiogenic shock causing poor cardiac output:
  - Myocardial infarction
  - Congestive cardiac failure
- Vasogenic shock:
  - Sepsis
  - Anaphylaxis
  - Neurogenic shock
  - Medications: vasodilation agents, anaesthetic agents
- Obstructive shock:
  - Constructive pericarditis
  - Cardiac tamponade
  - Pulmonary embolism

- Reduced renal perfusion:
  - Renovascular disease, e.g. renal artery or renal vein occlusion secondary to thrombosis or stenosis
  - Noradrenaline, adrenaline
  - Aortic dissection
  - Eclampsia (in setting of pregnancy)

Renal causes:

- Acute tubular necrosis
- Glomerulonephritis
- Interstitial nephritis
- Rhabdomyolysis

Post-renal causes:

- Upper renal tract obstruction
- Lower urinary tract obstruction:
  - Prostatic enlargement
  - Tumour
  - Stones
- Extrinsic compression of renal tract, e.g. intra-abdominal
- Blocked urinary indwelling catheter (IDC), if present

Before starting

Establish rapport:

- Introduce yourself
- Obtain consent from the patient: "I will be asking you some questions and then will be

performing a physical examination to find out why you have low urine output. Is this OK with you?"

- Expose the patient: when physical examination is required

Confirm patient details:
- Name   *Sean Mcmean*
- Age   *67 years*
- Occupation   *School teacher*

History

What is the reason for admission?

- *This patient had an emergency appendicectomy after presenting with abdominal pain*
- *An IDC was placed pre-operatively*

Associated symptoms

- *Abdominal pain (particularly in the suprapubic area) especially when trying to pass urine*
- Dysuria: *yes*
- Fever / chills / rigors: *yes, overnight*
- Sensation of thirst: *yes*
- Shortness of breath, peripheral oedema: *no*
- Paraesthesia / anaesthesia, especially saddle region: *normal*

Past medical history and family history

- Baseline renal function: *estimated glomerular filtration rate (eGFR) 60*
- *Type 2 diabetes mellitus, congestive cardiac failure, hypertension*
- *Known benign prostatic hypertrophy; no history of prostate cancer / treatment to prostate (such as radiotherapy, surgery)*
- *No history of renal stones or bladder tumours*
- *Nil family history*

Drug history and allergies

- *Aspirin, furosemide, irbesartan*
- *Recent IV contrast: the patient had a contrast CT abdomen / pelvis scan performed 1 day prior to the operation*
- *NKDA*

Social history

- Smoking history: *20 pack-years*
- Alcohol and drugs history: *non-drinker, nil illicit drugs*
- *Independent with daily activities; home with wife*

Examination

General inspection (ABCD-V)

- **A**ppearance: *alert, looks tired*
- **B**ody habitus: *obese, BMI 31*
- **C**ognition: *patient is conscious and oriented*
- **D**evices / **D**rugs:
  - *The patient is not using supplemental oxygen*
  - *IV fluids are running at a 12-hourly rate*
  - *IDC in situ, small amount of concentrated urine in the bag; no erythema / irritation at the external urethral meatus*
  - *Not on dialysis*
- **V**itals: *BP 90/60mmHg, HR 110bpm, RR 20 per minute; oxygen saturation at 95% on room air; febrile 38°C*

Fluid review

- Check perfusion of peripheries (*normal*), tissue turgor (*slow*)
- Check jugular venous pressure (*not elevated*), mucous membranes (*dry*)
- Listen to heart and chest (*heart sounds dual, nil added; chest is clear*)
- *No evidence of peripheral and sacral oedema*
- Review of fluid balance charts (fluid input and output): *negative balance over past day*

Abdomen

- Inspection:
  - Previous surgical scars or abnormalities: *no*
  - Signs of liver disease, e.g caput medusae, spider naevi, gynaecomastia: *no*
  - *The patient is not overtly distended in the abdomen*
- Palpation:
  - *The patient is tender to palpation in the suprapubic region*
  - Hepatosplenomegaly: *no*
- Percussion:
  - Dullness: *no, normal resonant sounds*
  - Ascites: *no*
- Auscultation:
  - Bowel sounds: *normal*
  - Renal artery bruits: *no*

Investigations

BBMI-O: Bedside, **B**loods, **M**icrobiology, **I**maging and **O**ther

Investigation	Rationale
Bedside	
▩ Urine dipstick	▩ Looking for infection (leukocytes, nitrites for pyelonephritis)
▩ Bladder scan	▩ Assessing if urinary retention is present – bladder volume
▩ ECG	▩ Perform if potassium is elevated above normal, for ECG changes related to hyperkalaemia (K$^+$ >5.5); or if there is reason to suspect a cardiogenic source for low urine output
Bloods	
▩ FBC	▩ Looking for infection
▩ U&Es and creatinine + eGFR	▩ Looking at electrolytes and renal function
▩ Venous blood gas	▩ Looking at electrolyte balance
▩ CRP	▩ Can be useful in the setting of infection
▩ Troponin I	▩ If suspicious of myocardial infarction
Microbiology	
▩ Urine MCS	▩ Looking for infection
▩ Other cultures as appropriate, e.g. blood cultures, sputum MCS	
Imaging	
▩ CXR	▩ Assess for fluid status, lung field consolidation
▩ Renal tract US	▩ Looking for hydronephrosis and other abnormalities in the renal tract
▩ CT urography	▩ Looking for stones in the renal tract; imaging may also visualise inflammatory changes secondary to infection (e.g. pyelonephritis)
Other	

Diagnosis

Poor urine output in the setting of urinary tract infection / sepsis

A patient with an IDC pre-op that now presents with fevers, dysuria and clinical dehydration is highly suggestive.

Management

Medical

- Review medication chart for nephrotoxins and rationalise / cease those possible
- Supplemental IV fluids may be of benefit in hypovolaemia, but ensure other causes are ruled out to ensure that the patient is not being overloaded with fluid
- Completing a septic screen and commencing IV antibiotics can be considered in the setting of infection

- Consider flushing or changing an IDC if required (e.g. in the context of a blocked IDC)

Surgical

- Not indicated in this case
- Applicable in cases of post-renal obstruction (i.e. stones) causing the oliguria

Other differential diagnoses

- Nephrolithiasis
- Hypovolaemia

Station 52 **Palpitations**

A 40-year-old woman presents to the GP complaining of several episodes of palpitations.

Tasks

1 Take a history
2 Perform a targeted examination

3 Describe appropriate investigations
4 Formulate a management plan

Differential diagnoses (VIITAMINC)

Vascular:
- Valvular heart disease, prosthetic heart valves
- Cardiac and extracardiac shunts
- Arrhythmia
- Cardiomyopathy
- Atrial myxoma
- Anaemia

Infective:
- Fever

Inflammatory

Trauma

Autoimmune

Metabolic:
- Hypoglycaemia
- Hyperthyroidism, thyrotoxicosis

Iatrogenic:
- Pacemaker-related tachycardia

- Drug-induced – sympathomimetics, vasodilators, anticholinergics, beta-blocker withdrawal, benzodiazepine withdrawal, caffeine, energy drinks, weight loss medications, nicotine, cannabis, cocaine, amphetamines

Neoplastic:
- Phaeochromocytoma

Congenital

Other:
- Pregnancy
- Postural orthostatic tachycardia syndrome
- Stress, exercise
- Panic attacks
- Generalised anxiety disorder
- Somatisation
- Depression

Before starting

Establish rapport:
- Introduce yourself
- Obtain consent from the patient: "I will be asking you some questions and then will be performing a physical examination to find out why you have palpitations. Is this OK with you?"

- Expose the patient: when physical examination is required

Confirm patient details:
- Name   *Cassandra Clarke*
- Age   *40 years*
- Occupation   *Magazine editor*

History

History regarding palpitations

- Site: *over the chest*
- Quality:
  - Regular / irregular: *irregular*
  - Skipping beats / feeling that heartbeat stops: *no*
  - Sensation of the palpitations: *flutter sensation and sometimes it feels as though heart is racing*
- Time course:
  - Onset: *abrupt, this morning*
  - Offset: *none, as of yet*
  - Duration: *4 hours*
  - Frequency: *random, a few episodes a year*
  - Constant or episodic in nature: *episodic*
- Context: *no particular context*
- Aggravating factors: *worsens with excessive alcohol consumption*
- Relieving factors: *nil specific*
- Associated symptoms: *yes, feels short of breath and has some chest pain when the episodes occur*

Past medical history and family history

- *Nil significant past medical history*
- *Maternal aunt had thyroid disease with a heart condition*

Drug history and allergies

- *Nil*
- *NKDA*

Social history:

- Smoking history: *20 pack-years*
- Alcohol and drugs history: *2 drinks per day, binges on weekends, occasional cannabis use*

Examination

General inspection (ABCD-V)

- **A**ppearance: *patient looks comfortable*
- **B**ody habitus: *normal, BMI 21*
- **C**ognition: *conscious and oriented*
- **D**evices / **D**rugs: *none*
- **V**itals: *BP 110/70mmHg, HR 115bpm, RR 20 per minute; oxygen saturation at 97% on room air; afebrile*

Neck examination

- Thyroid examination:
  - Inspection: *normal, no goitre*
  - Palpation: *palpable thyroid gland, no goitre or lumps*
  - Percussion: *no retrosternal dullness*
  - Auscultation: *no thyroid bruit*
- Lymphadenopathy: *none detected*
- Trachea: *midline*

Cardiovascular examination

- Hands:
  - Assess hands for evidence of increased sweating, palmar erythema, tremor: *none*
  - Pulse: *radial pulse is strong, though irregularly irregular rhythm and tachycardic; no radial-radial delay*
  - BP: *no significant postural drop*
- Chest:
  - Inspection: *normal, no surgical scars or abnormalities; no obvious pacemaker visible; no clubbing or stigmata of peripheral endocarditis; jugular venous pressure not elevated (+2cm)*
  - Palpation: *apex palpable at 5th intercostal space, mid-clavicular line; no palpable heave or thrill*
  - Auscultation:
    - Dual heart sounds, loss of S4; irregularly irregular contractions
    - No pleural rub or pericardial rub
  - Assess for pacemaker placement: *none*

Neurological examination

- Inspection: *normal*
- Reflexes, tone, power and sensation: *normal*

Investigations

BBMI-O: Bedside, **B**loods, **M**icrobiology, **I**maging and **O**ther

Investigation	Rationale
Bedside	
12-lead ECG	Tachycardia – check if sinus tachycardia; assess for arrhythmia
Bloods	
FBC, TFTs (TSH, T_3, T_4)	Limited laboratory testing to rule out anaemia and hyperthyroidism is reasonable, in addition to testing for specific disorders that may be suggested by the history and physical examination
Specific thyroid autoimmune blood tests: TSI, TSH receptor Ab, anti-TPO Ab	If suspicious for Graves' disease
U&Es and creatinine, CMP for potassium and magnesium can be useful for patients with AF	Aim to optimise $K^+ >4$, $Mg^{2+} >1$
Troponin I (± repeat in 6 hours' time for trend)	Only for patients who have palpitations and suspected coronary ischaemia
Microbiology	
Appropriate specimens could be sent for analysis if suspecting infection and a potential source (e.g. in a febrile patient)	
Imaging	
US	To assess size, echotexture and vascularity
Nuclear medicine uptake scans, e.g. ^{99m}Tc pertechnetate, ^{123}I	To assess for homogenously increased activity in an enlarged thyroid gland
Echocardiography	To assess for structural heart disease
Other (for other causes of palpitations)	
Ambulatory monitoring (Holter monitor, continuous loop event recorder)	For definitive diagnosis of palpitations secondary to arrhythmia

Investigation	Rationale
Exercise stress testing	To provoke exercise-induced palpitations
Interrogation of implanted cardiac devices	To see if arrhythmia has been documented on certain devices
Urine screening when appropriate: metanephrine and electrolyte levels; urine drug screen	

Diagnosis

Atrial fibrillation (AF)

A history of fluttering palpitations that worsens with alcohol intake in a patient that examines benignly is suspicious for paroxysmal AF.

Management

Medical

- Rate control: beta-blockers (i.e. metoprolol), calcium channel blockers (CCBs, e.g. diltiazem, verapamil; in patients with heart failure: digoxin, amiodarone)
  - Don't give beta-blocker and central CCB together – bradycardia risk
- Rhythm control: pharmacological cardioversion: flecainide first choice if no structural disease (IV amiodarone if disease present), sotalol
- Anticoagulation: warfarin, dabigatran, rivaroxaban, apixaban – thromboembolism prevention (4% per year)
- Cardioversion (electrical):
  - If symptomatic <24–48h usually cardiovert without anticoagulation

- If symptomatic >24–48h anticoagulate for 3 weeks prior and 4 weeks post
- If patient unstable: cardiovert immediately
- Aetiology: treat the underlying cause if possible
- Paroxysmal AF: pill in pocket (sotalol or flecainide PRN) and anticoagulate

Surgical

- MAZE: surgical ablation, use of small incisions, radiowaves or freezing to create scar tissue which does not conduct electrical activity

Other differential diagnoses

- Hypoglycaemia
- Amphetamines

Station 53 **Paraesthesia**

A 40-year-old woman presents to the GP complaining of numbness and tingling and pain in part of her right hand.

Tasks

1 Take a history
2 Perform a targeted examination
3 Describe appropriate investigations
4 Formulate a management plan

Differential diagnoses (VIITAMINC)

Vascular:
- Peripheral vascular disease
- Stroke

Infective

Inflammatory:
- Carpal tunnel syndrome
- Medial or ulnar neuropathy
- Fibular neuropathy
- Radiculopathy
- Plexopathy

Trauma:
- Vertebral disc herniation

Autoimmune:
- Rheumatoid arthritis
- Demyelinating conditions (e.g. multiple sclerosis)
- Guillain–Barré syndrome

Metabolic:
- Vitamin deficiencies, e.g. B_6, B_{12}
- Hypothyroidism
- Diabetes mellitus
- Hypocalcaemia
- Uraemia

Iatrogenic:
- Medication-related, e.g. amiodarone, statins, anti-retrovirals, tacrolimus, chemotherapeutics
- Radiation-related

Neoplastic:
- Central nervous system malignancy

Congenital

Other:
- Fibromyalgia
- Migraine with aura
- Panic attack with hyperventilation

Before starting

Establish rapport:
- Introduce yourself
- Obtain consent from the patient: "I will be asking you some questions and then will be performing a physical examination to find out why you have a change in sensation. Is this OK with you?"

- Expose the patient: when physical examination is required

Confirm patient details:
- Name   *Lucy Cook*
- Age   *40 years*
- Occupation   *Secretary*

History

Regarding paraesthesia

- Site: *paraesthesia in the right hand, affecting lateral part of the hand, including the lateral three and a half digits, but sparing the thenar eminence*
- Quality: *pins and needles sensation*
- Severity: *affects her work duties – heavy typist*
- Time course:
  - Onset: *gradual*
  - Offset: *gradual (with rest)*
  - Duration: *lasts with duration of repetitive activity or awkward positioning, but seems to be random at times as of late*
  - Frequency: *often*
- Aggravating factors: *repetitive actions that involve her right hand*
- Relieving factors: *rest of right hand; sometimes shaking the right hand / upper limb helps*
- Context: *no history of trauma; can occur at work with repetitive actions; symptoms overall flared up during her pregnancy 2 years ago*
- Associated symptoms:
  - *Dull, aching pain in right hand: worse at night; shooting sensation of pain from the wrist at times*
  - *Weakness and clumsiness of the right hand has occurred previously*
- Dominant hand: *right-handed*

Past medical history and family history

- *Type 2 diabetes mellitus*
- *Nil family history*

Drug history and allergies

- *Metformin 500mg BD*
- *NKDA*

Social history

- Smoking history: *non-smoker*
- Alcohol and drugs history: *social drinker, nil illicit drugs*

Examination

General inspection (ABCD-V)

- **A**ppearance: *looks well*
- **B**ody habitus: *obese, BMI 34*
- **C**ognition: *normal*
- **D**evices / **D**rugs: *none*
- **V**itals: *all within normal limits*

Neurological examination

- Inspection: *normal orientation of the upper limbs; no skin changes evident*
- Tone: *normal tone*
- Power: *normal*
- Reflexes: *normal upper limb reflexes*
- Sensation: *mildly reduced in median nerve distribution of the hand, but sensation in the thenar eminence is normal*

Neck examination

- Inspect: *no abnormality evident*
- Palpation of the cervical spine: *no midline tenderness*
- *Normal neck range of motion*

A full back examination could be appropriate if the concern was related to potential nerve issues at other vertebral levels.

Other tests

- Tinel's test: *negative*
- Phalen's test: *positive*

Investigations

BBMI-O: Bloods, **M**icrobiology, **I**maging and **O**ther

Investigation	Rationale
Bedside	
Bloods	
Vitamin B$_{12}$, magnesium	For other causes of muscle cramping / pain sensation
HbA1c	To review control of diabetes
Microbiology	
Imaging	
X-ray of hand / wrist	Relevant if suspicious of trauma to the hand in a more acute situation; to rule out a fracture
US or MRI of the hand / wrist	May be useful to evaluate for structural abnormality of the wrist, e.g. tumour, deformity, or other bone and joint disease
Other	
Neurophysiology studies, e.g. nerve conduction studies and EMG	Can be supplementary to diagnosing carpal tunnel syndrome (primarily a clinical diagnosis); has high sensitivity and specificity for confirming the diagnosis, and can gauge severity of median nerve injury and exclude other diagnoses in the differential diagnosis

Diagnosis

Carpal tunnel syndrome

An obese patient with an occupation requiring heavy typing with positive Phalen's test and median nerve symptoms is typical of carpal tunnel syndrome.

Management

Supportive
- Rest
- Physiotherapy
- Supportive splints – especially at night

Medical
- Diuresis if secondary to oedema
- Local anaesthetic into the carpal tunnel
- Corticosteroid injections into the carpal tunnel

Surgical
- Carpal tunnel release procedure

Other differential diagnoses

- Cervical radiculopathy (particularly with C6 or C7 nerve root involvement)

Station 54 **Polyuria**

A 35-year-old woman presents with increased voiding of urine volume and urinary frequency.

Tasks

1 Take a history
2 Perform a targeted examination
3 Describe appropriate investigations
4 Formulate a management plan

Differential diagnoses

- Diabetes mellitus (DM)
- Diabetes insipidus (DI)
- Medication- or substance-related
  - Diuretics, mannitol
  - Lithium toxicity, amphotericin B (nephrogenic DI)
  - Caffeine, ethanol
- Renal disease (inability to reabsorb water)
  - Diuretic phase of acute tubular necrosis

- Post-obstructive diuresis
- Salt-losing nephritis
- Polycystic kidney disease (nephrogenic DI)
- Physiological diuresis
  - For example, secondary to increased glomerular filtration rate in hyperthyroidism, fever, hypermetabolic states

---

Before starting

Establish rapport:
- Introduce yourself
- Obtain consent from the patient: "I will be asking you some questions and then will be performing a physical examination to find out why you have high urine output. Is this OK with you?"
- Expose the patient: when physical examination is required

Confirm patient details:
- Name   *Claire Short*
- Age   *35 years*
- Occupation   *Homemaker*

History

Symptoms related to polyuria

- Time course:
  - Duration: *a few days*
  - Onset: *sudden, 1–2 weeks ago* (often gradual in acquired nephrogenic DI or primary polydipsia)
- Offset: *ongoing*
- Frequency: *increased urinary frequency throughout the day; new nocturia, with production of non-concentrated urine in high volumes overnight and in early morning*
- Amount of fluid intake for the patient per day: *feels thirsty so has needed to increase fluid intake accordingly to >5L per day*
- Severity: *affecting sleep as needing to rouse often to urinate*
- Aggravating and relieving factors: *none clear*
- Context: *recent surgery to pituitary gland 1 month ago*

Associated symptoms

- *No symptoms of urinary tract infection including dysuria / lower urinary tract symptoms (e.g. urgency)*
- *Sensation of thirst*
- Loss of weight (can occur in diabetes mellitus due to loss of glucose): *a few kilograms*
- *Complains of peripheral vision loss (reason why she presented), dull headache not resolving with simple analgesia*

Past medical history and family history

- Nil significant past medical history
- Nil family history

Drug history and allergies

- Nil
- NKDA

Social history

- Smoking history: 10 pack-years
- Alcohol and drugs history: non-drinker, nil illicit drugs

Examination

General inspection (ABCD-V)

- **A**ppearance: patient is comfortable
- **B**ody habitus: obese, BMI 32
- **C**ognition: normal, alert and oriented
- **D**evices / **D**rugs: nil
- **V**itals: BP 135/80mmHg, HR 95bpm, RR 16 per minute; oxygen saturation at 97% on room air; afebrile

Appearance of urine in collection bottle: appears dilute

Fluid review

- Check perfusion of peripheries (normal), tissue turgor (slow)
- Check jugular venous pressure (not elevated), mucous membranes (dry)
- Listen to heart and chest (heart sounds dual, nil added; chest is clear)
- No evidence of peripheral and sacral oedema
- Review of fluid balance charts (fluid input and output): increased oral fluid intake and urine output

Neurological examination

- Eye examination yields a bitemporal hemianopia; normal visual acuity
- Normal neurological examination otherwise

Other

- Abdomen: soft, non-tender
- Signs of anaemia (can occur in chronic kidney disease): none
- Fundus examination in DM (normal), hypertension for papilloedema (present)

Investigations

BBMI-O: Bedside, **B**loods, **M**icrobiology, **I**maging and **O**ther

Investigation	Rationale
Bedside	
Urine dipstick	Rule out infection given associated urinary frequency; send urine for MCS if positive for infection (leukocytes, nitrites)
Bloods	
U&Es and creatinine	Serum sodium level, renal function
Plasma osmolality	To compare with urine osmolality to determine concentrations
Microbiology	
Imaging	
US renal tract	Can help establish diagnosis of polycystic kidney disease

Investigation	Rationale
Other	
▓ 24-hour urine collection – urine osmolality	▓ Can be difficult for the patient but can allow calculation of 24-hour urine osmolality, to measure the ability for the kidneys to concentrate urine
▓ Water deprivation test	▓ For evaluation of DI; involves complete fluid deprivation, and administration of hypertonic NaCl solution and exogenous ADH, with measurement of the ADH to serum osmolality ratio

Diagnosis

Central diabetes insipidus (DI) secondary to pituitary adenoma

A patient that presents with polyuria and is clinically dehydrated, with a bitemporal hemianopia, likely suggests a pituitary origin of polyuria.

Discussion

▓ Primary polydipsia (also called psychogenic polydipsia): a primary increase in daily water intake >6L per day

▓ Central DI – associated with deficient antidiuretic hormone (ADH) secretion, due to causes that affect ADH synthesis, transport or release:
  - Idiopathic (possibly autoimmune injury to ADH-producing cells)
  - Secondary to trauma, pituitary surgery, tumours, hypoxic ischaemic brain injury, inflammatory or infective brain conditions, vascular disease

▓ Nephrogenic DI – associated with normal ADH secretion but varying degrees of renal resistance to its water-retaining effect:

  - Can be caused by:
    ▹ Hypercalcaemia
    ▹ Hypokalaemia

▓ DI – high–normal plasma sodium concentration with urine osmolality less than that of plasma:
  - DI is excluded if: there is a normal sodium plasma concentration associated with a urinary osmolality more than 600mOsm/kg
  - In comparison, water overload secondary to primary polydipsia: low plasma sodium concentration with low urine osmolality (half that of plasma osmolality)

Other differential diagnoses

▓ Diabetes mellitus

Station 55 **Pruritus**

A 65-year-old man presents to the emergency department with a 2-week history of jaundice and itch.

Tasks

1 Take a history

2 Perform a targeted examination

3 Describe appropriate investigations

4 Formulate a management plan

Differential diagnoses (VIITAMINC)

Vascular

Infective:
- Scabies
- HIV

Inflammatory:
- Dermatitis (atopic, contact)
- Urticaria
- Dermatophytosis
- Lichen simplex
- Bullous pemphigoid

Trauma

Autoimmune:
- Psoriasis

Metabolic:
- Renal disease – secondary to uraemia
- Cholestasis
- Thyroid dysfunction

Iatrogenic:
- Medication-related

Neoplastic:
- Malignancy – particular haematological

Congenital:
- Connective tissue diseases

Other:
- Neurological disorders
- Psychogenic disorders

Before starting

Establish rapport:
- Introduce yourself
- Obtain consent from the patient: "I will be asking you some questions and then will be performing a physical examination to find out why you have an itch. Is this OK with you?"
- Expose the patient: when physical examination is required

Confirm patient details:
- Name   *Harry Seabrook*
- Age   *65 years*
- Occupation   *Retired office worker*

History

History of presenting complaint
- Site of itch: *generalised, began in palms and soles*
- Onset: *gradual onset; present for 1–2 weeks; first incidence of this problem*
- Severity of pruritus: *irritating during day; worse at night*
- *No obvious rash on skin*
- *Associated yellowing (jaundice) of face, sclera and peripheries noted by wife*

- Associated symptoms:
  - *Upper abdominal pain (constant dull ache in right upper quadrant, RUQ)*
  - *Subjective report of fevers, night sweats*
  - *Recent unintentional loss of weight (5–8kg) over 6 months*
  - *Feels tired*
  - *Mild nausea*
  - *Pale urine*
  - *Dark stools*
- Exacerbating / relieving factors: *no real exacerbating / relieving factors for the itch*

Past medical history and family history

- *Hypertension, type 2 diabetes mellitus, gout, psoriasis*
- *Nil family history*

Drug history and allergies

- *Medications: perindopril, metformin, gliclazide, allopurinol, topical corticosteroid*
- *Allergies: penicillin (rash)*

Social history

- Smoking history: *15 pack-years*
- Alcohol and drugs history: *2–3 drinks per day, nil illicit drugs*
- *Home with wife*
- *Independent with daily activities*

Examination

General inspection (ABCD-V)

- **A**ppearance: *looks uncomfortable*
- **B**ody habitus: *normal, BMI 24*
- **C**ognition: *normal, alert and oriented*
- **D**evices / **D**rugs: *none*
- **V**itals: *BP 140/90mmHg, HR 95bpm, RR 18 per minute; oxygen saturation at 96% on room air; afebrile*

Inspection of peripheries

- *Yellowing of palms*
- *Scleral icterus present*
- *No obvious rash on body or other peripheral stigmata of chronic liver disease, but some excoriation marks where patient states he has been itchy*
- *Patient appears euvolaemic*

Abdominal examination

- Inspection: *no previous abdominal surgery scars; not distended; mild yellow tinge to skin overall*
- Palpation: *tender in epigastrium and RUQ on palpation, but soft enlarged liver span 16cm, no splenomegaly; no inguinal lymphadenopathy noted*
- Percussion: *not peritonitic; no ascites of shifting dullness*
- Auscultation: *bowel sounds present*

Investigations

BBMI-O: Bedside, **B**loods, **M**icrobiology, **I**maging and **O**ther

Investigation	Rationale
Bedside	
Bloods	
FBC, U&Es and creatinine	Looking for anaemia, infection and electrolyte imbalances
LFTs (including ALP and direct, indirect and total bilirubin)	Elevated total bilirubin, direct bilirubin and ALP suggest extrahepatic cholangiocarcinoma; chronic biliary obstruction can cause generalised deranged LFTs
Coagulation profile	Ensure no coagulopathy is present in the setting of LFT derangement; patient may have an elevated INR and partial prothrombin time (PTT)
Tumour markers (e.g. CA 19-9)	May be elevated

Investigation	Rationale
Microbiology	
Blood cultures (peripheral)	To rule out bacteraemia, preferably taken prior to antibiotic commencement if patient stable
Imaging	
US abdomen	To confirm biliary duct dilatation, site of obstruction, and exclude gallstones
CT/MRI abdomen	If US is unable to confirm a benign cause of biliary obstruction as a cause of jaundice
Endoscopic US or ERCP	For next step in evaluation of extrahepatic cholangiocarcinoma; endoscopic US could enable a biopsy; ERCP could potentiate stent placement
Other	

Diagnosis

Obstructive jaundice secondary to malignant biliary obstruction (from extrahepatic cholangiocarcinoma)

This patient exhibits signs of jaundice and a non-tender RUQ mass with unintentional loss of weight, which are red flags for biliary malignancy.

Discussion

- A neoplasm of the biliary system, where 95% are adenocarcinomas arising from the epithelial cells within the biliary tree
- Courvoisier's law: presence of jaundice and a non-tender palpable RUQ mass is a biliary neoplasm until proven otherwise

Management

Medical

- Antihistamine: symptom reduction
- Cholestyramine: increases biliary drainage
- Analgesia as required
- Radiotherapy: adjunct or neoadjunct therapy to lessen the tumour size

Surgical

- Tumour resection: to lessen the tumour compression/occlusion of the common hepatic duct, though majority of patients (85–90%) are deemed inoperable at time of presentation

Palliative

- Stenting via endoscopic retrograde cholangiopancreatography (ERCP): to relieve obstructive symptoms
- Surgical bypass: management of obstruction if stenting fails
- Chemoradiotherapy: to prolong survival

Other differential diagnoses

- Eczema (atopic dermatitis)
- Medication-induced

Station 56 **Rectal bleeding**

A 72-year-old woman with a known history of diverticulosis presents to the emergency department with rectal bleeding.

Tasks

1 Take a history
2 Perform a targeted examination
3 Describe appropriate investigations
4 Formulate a management plan

Differential diagnoses

Upper gastrointestinal (GI) bleeding:
- Peptic ulcer disease
- Gastric erosion / stress ulcers
- Mallory–Weiss tear
- Oesophageal varices
- Oesophagitis
- Gastritis
- Malignancy
- Angiodysplasia (vascular malformation)
- Trauma
- Iatrogenic

Lower GI bleeding:
- Diverticulosis
- Colitis
  - Inflammatory

- Infectious
- Ischaemic
- Inflammatory bowel disease
- Colonic malignancy or polyp
- Mesenteric ischaemia
- Angiodysplasia
- Congenital
  - Meckel's diverticulum
- Anorectal conditions
  - Haemorrhoids
  - Anal fissure
- Aorto-enteric fistula
- Trauma
- Iatrogenic, e.g. postoperative, post-biopsy / polypectomy

Before starting

Establish rapport:
- Introduce yourself
- Obtain consent from the patient: "I will be asking you some questions and then will be performing a physical examination including a digital rectal examination, to find out why you have rectal bleeding. Is this OK with you?"
- Expose the patient: when physical examination is required
- Ensure a chaperone is present during the examination

Confirm patient details:
- Name   *Isla O'Hare*
- Age   *72 years*
- Occupation   *Retired*

History

Nature of bleeding

- Duration, colour, amount of blood, mixed with stools or on paper / into toilet bowl:
  - *The patient thought they were attempting to open their bowels overnight, but instead had passage of a large amount of maroon-coloured blood and clots (likely >1 cup in amount in the toilet bowl); this was not mixed with stool*
- Frequency: *first episode*
- Time of onset, progression:
  - *Sudden onset*

- The patient has not attempted to open their bowels again post this issue; however, feels some urgency to do so
- Associated pain, site (abdomen, anal orifice, etc.) and occurrence:
  - The patient experienced severe cramping left lower abdominal pain before attempting to use the toilet; the cramping pain was somewhat relieved post passage of the blood motion
- Associated symptoms (e.g. febrile illness, retching preceding haematemesis, anaemia, change in bowel habit, distension, weight loss):
  - The patient had cramping left lower abdominal pain for the last 1–2 days
  - Associated nausea, no vomiting, mild loss of appetite
  - Felt hot, but no measured fevers
- Bowel habits (e.g. constipation versus diarrhoea), and if any change has occurred recently:
  - The patient had last opened their bowels 2 days ago (diarrhoea); usually fluctuates between constipation and diarrhoea but opens bowels on average every 1–2 days

Past medical history and family history

- Atrial fibrillation, hypertension, type 2 diabetes mellitus
- Open appendicectomy in childhood for perforated appendicitis
- Previous colonoscopy 3 years ago post episode of diverticulitis; confirmed severe sigmoid diverticulosis, no polyps
- Mother had bowel cancer

Drug history and allergies

- Irbesartan, metformin, apixaban
- NKDA

Social history

- Smoking history: 25 pack-years
- Alcohol and drugs history: non-drinker, nil illicit drugs
- Home alone, mobilises with 4-wheel frame

Examination

General inspection (ABCD-V)

- **A**ppearance: looks tired
- **B**ody habitus: obese, BMI 31
- **C**ognition: sleepy, but Glasgow Coma Score (GCS) 15
- **D**evices / **D**rugs: IV fluids running at 10-hourly rate in one arm; no indwelling catheter in situ
- **V**itals: BP 100/60mmHg, HR 100bpm, RR 22 per minute; oxygen saturation at 96% on room air; low-grade temperature 37.7°C

Fluid review

- Check perfusion of peripheries (normal), tissue turgor (slow)
- Check jugular venous pressure (not elevated), mucous membranes (dry)
- Listen to heart and chest (heart sounds dual, nil added; chest is clear)
- No evidence of peripheral and sacral oedema

Abdominal examination

- Inspection:
  - Mildly distended abdomen
  - Previous appendicectomy scar on right lower quadrant
- Palpation:
  - Tender in the left iliac fossa; remaining abdomen is soft
  - No hepatosplenomegaly
- Percussion:
  - No peritonitis
  - No ascites
- Auscultation:
  - Slow bowel sounds

Per rectal (PR) examination (with consent + chaperone)

- Assess anal orifice for signs of haemorrhoids, anal fissure, any other obvious abnormalities: no inflammatory skin changes, tags or masses noted
- Digital rectal examination with gloved finger and lubricant; palpable masses or abnormalities, pain on examination: normal rectal mucosa
- On withdrawal from rectal examination, examine gloved finger for colour of any blood, stool appearance, odour: maroon blood on glove, no frank red blood

Investigations

BBMI-O: Bedside, **B**loods, **M**icrobiology, **I**maging and **O**ther

Investigation	Rationale
Bedside	
Bloods	
▦ FBE	▦ Check Hb, check WCC for signs of infection, check platelets for clotting ability
▦ U&Es and creatinine	▦ Check renal function, check urea for suspicion of upper GI bleeding
▦ LFTs	▦ Check liver function as abnormality raises the risk of underlying severe liver disease and thus coagulopathy and varices
▦ CRP	▦ Can check if suspecting an infective cause
▦ Coagulation profile	▦ Check INR, activated partial thromboplastin time (APTT)
▦ Group and hold ± cross-match	▦ In case of requiring transfusion
Microbiology	
▦ Stool MCS + *Clostridium difficile* toxin	▦ If presenting with diarrhoea (e.g. secondary to colitis)
Imaging	
▦ Erect CXR	▦ Useful to assess for free gas under the diaphragm if patient has abdominal tenderness secondary to a perforated viscus
▦ CT angiography	▦ To see if there is active bleeding with view of management planning (embolisation, surgery, monitoring); requires bleeding at a rate of approximately 0.5ml/min to detect active bleeding
▦ Red cell scan (nuclear medicine)	▦ To see if there is active bleeding with view of management planning (embolisation, surgery, monitoring); can be more useful if per rectal bleeding is at a slower rate (as slow as 0.05ml/min), but this scan takes time and is not easy to complete in an urgent setting
Other	
▦ Endoscopy (gastroscopy / colonoscopy)	▦ To directly visualise any abnormalities causing acute bleeding

---

Diagnosis

Diverticular bleed (concurrent diverticulitis)

A patient with known history of diverticular disease that presents with acute PR bleeding and low-grade fever is suggestive of diverticulitis.

Discussion

- Outpouching of the bowel mucosa in weakened areas (diverticulosis) which can become inflamed / infected (diverticulitis)
- Complications that can occur include pericolic abscess, fistula formation and bowel obstruction
- Uncomplicated diverticulitis: localised diverticulitis
- Complicated diverticulitis: diverticulitis associated with complications, including the presence of rectal bleeding, abscess, fistula, obstruction or perforation

Management

Medical

- Analgesia as required
- IV fluid replacement: resuscitation and maintenance
- Bowel rest: clear fluids only
- IV antibiotics: gentamicin (or piperacillin + tazobactam beyond 72 hours of IV antibiotics) + amoxycillin / ampicillin + metronidazole; downgrade to oral once patient has been afebrile for 24–48 hours
- Blood transfusion: in cases with significant PR haemorrhage

Surgical

- Required in 15–30% of admitted patients
- If active rectal bleeding: colonoscopy for endoscopic haemostasis if appropriate
- Peritoneal washout ± bowel resection (Hartmann's)
- Emergency surgery (laparoscopy or laparotomy): in cases of perforation with faecal peritonitis or overwhelming sepsis
- Urgent surgery (laparoscopy or laparotomy): in cases where medical management has failed or the patient required percutaneous drainage (complication with perforation or abscess)

Other differential diagnoses

- Haemorrhoids

Station 57 **Scrotal mass**

A 45-year-old man presents to the emergency department with a scrotal mass.

Tasks

1 Take a history
2 Perform a targeted examination
3 Describe appropriate investigations
4 Formulate a management plan

Differential diagnoses (VIITAMINC)

Vascular

Infective:
- Epididymo-orchitis

Inflammatory:
- Sebaceous cyst
- Scrotal oedema
- Hydrocele
- Varicocele
- Spermatocele
- Testicular torsion
- Torsion of testicular appendage

Trauma:
- Haematocele

Autoimmune

Metabolic

Iatrogenic

Neoplastic:
- Squamous cell carcinoma
- Testicular tumour
- Epididymal cyst

Congenital:
- Indirect inguinal hernia

Other

Before starting

Establish rapport:
- Introduce yourself
- Obtain consent from the patient: "I'll be asking you questions then perform a physical exam to clarify the cause of your scrotal mass / swelling. Is this OK with you?"
- Expose the patient: when physical examination is required

Confirm patient details:
- Name   *John James*
- Age   *45 years*
- Occupation   *Welder*

History

History of presenting complaint
- Specific site of problem: *right testicle*
- Severity + quality of the swelling / mass: *hard lump approximately 1.5 × 2cm, otherwise normal*
- Time course of problem:
  - Onset (gradual versus sudden): *noticed 2 months ago, though gradual increase in size*
  - Duration: *2 months*
- Context: *first noticed when in the shower 2 months ago, no association to trauma*
- Exacerbating / relieving factors: *no*
- Associated symptoms:
  - *Painless lump, over the last week it has become a dull ache*

- Scrotal skin changes: *no*
- Nausea, vomiting, constitutional symptoms (e.g. unintentional loss of weight, fatigue, night sweats): *more tired than usual, otherwise normal*
- Lower urinary tract symptoms, e.g. frequency: *no*
- Abnormal penile discharge: *no*
- Infective symptoms: *no*

Past medical history and family history

- *Previous scrotal surgery including orchidopexy*
- *Mother had breast cancer at age 60 years, father has type 2 diabetes mellitus*

Drug history and allergies

- *Nil*
- *NKDA*

Social history

- Smoking history: *15 pack-years*
- Alcohol and drugs history: *2 drinks per day, nil illicit drugs*

Examination

General inspection (ABCD-V)

- **A**ppearance: *patient looks well*
- **B**ody habitus: *overweight, BMI 28*
- **C**ognition: *patient is conscious and oriented*
- **D**evices / **D**rugs: *no*
- **V**itals: *BP 130/85mmHg, HR 65bpm; oxygen saturation at 99% on room air; afebrile*

Abdominal examination

- Inspection: *no surgical scars, deformities or visible pulsations are noted on the abdomen*
- Palpation: *no tenderness, no hepatosplenomegaly*
- Percussion: *no percussive peritonitis, no ascites*
- Auscultation: *normal bowel sounds*

Focused scrotal examination

- Obtain consent from the patient to complete this part of the examination
- Adequate exposure: ensure that the patient is comfortable and ask them to change into a gown or to undress and cover their lower half with a blanket prior to your examination of the scrotum
- Characteristics of describing an area of mass or swelling:
  - Site: *right testicle*
  - Size: *2cm × 2cm*
  - Tenderness: *no*
  - Irregular / smooth: *irregular*
  - Solid / soft / fluctuant: *solid*
  - Can the borders of the mass or swelling be palpated: *no*
  - Transilluminescence: *no*
  - Scrotal appearance: *normal*
  - Auscultation (if suspecting indirect inguinal hernia): *no*
  - Cough impulse (if suspecting indirect inguinal hernia) – often useful to examine with the patient standing up: *no*
  - Inguinal lymphadenopathy (for superficial pathology): *no*

Investigations

BBMI-O: Bedside, **B**loods, **M**icrobiology, **I**maging and **O**ther

Investigation	Rationale
Bedside	
Bloods	
FBC	Looking for infection
CRP	Looking for infection
Alpha-fetoprotein, beta-hCG, LDH	Tumour markers

Investigation	Rationale
Microbiology	
Genital swab MCS	If there is evidence of penile discharge relating to possible infection
Imaging	
Testicular US	For characterisation of a lesion in the scrotum (e.g. solid, fluid)
Other	

Diagnosis

Testicular neoplasm (seminoma)

A painless, hard lump in a middle-aged man that examines unremarkably is testicular malignancy until proven otherwise.

Discussion

It is the most common malignancy in young men, with peak incidence 20–34 years of age.

Management

Medical

- Surveillance: only stage 1 disease, where the seminoma is confined to the testis / tunica vaginalis
- Radiation: for localised or low-volume seminomas
- Chemotherapy:
  - Seminoma: carboplatin
  - Non-seminoma (i.e. choriocarcinoma) or advanced seminomas: bleomycin, etoposide, cisplatin (BEP) combination

Surgical

- Radical inguinal orchiectomy: first-line treatment for a suspicious testicular mass; complete resection of the involved testicle, spermatic cord and appendages
- Retroperitoneal lymph node dissection (RLND): post orchiectomy in non-seminoma patients

Other differential diagnoses

- Indirect inguinal hernia
- Testicular torsion

Station 58 **Skin hyperpigmentation**

An 80-year-old Caucasian man presents with an irregular hyperpigmented lesion on his upper back, which was first pointed out by his wife.

Tasks

1 Take a history
2 Perform a targeted examination
3 Describe appropriate investigations
4 Formulate a management plan

Differential diagnoses (VIITAMINC)

Vascular

Infective

Inflammatory:
- Post-inflammatory hyperpigmentation
- Dermatosis papulosa nigra
- Melanosis (Becker's, smoker's)
- Primary cutaneous amyloidosis

Trauma

Autoimmune:
- Lichen planus

Metabolic:
- Addison's disease
- Diabetic dermopathy
- Acanthosis nigricans
- Hyperthyroidism

Iatrogenic:
- Fixed drug eruption
- Medication-induced diffuse hyperpigmentation

Neoplastic

Congenital:
- Congenital dermal melanocytosis
- Lentigines
- Hereditary haemochromatosis

Other:
- Ephelides (freckles)
- Melasma
- Acquired naevi (benign melanocytic naevus, atypical / dysplastic naevus, blue naevus)
- Maturational hyperpigmentation

Before starting

Establish rapport:
- Introduce yourself
- Obtain consent from the patient: "I'll be asking you questions then perform a physical exam to clarify the cause of your change in skin appearance / hyperpigmented skin lesion. Is this OK with you?"
- Expose the patient: when physical examination is required

Confirm patient details:
- Name — *James Woodson*
- Age — *80 years*
- Occupation — *Retired farmer*

History

ABCDE mnemonic for points to describe a lesion suspicious for melanoma:
- **A**symmetry: *asymmetrical across the two halves of the lesion*
- **B**orders: *irregular, uneven*

Colour: *multiple or changing shades of colour*

Diameter: *8 × 15mm*

Evolution: *first noticed this lesion 6 months ago, over time it has become more raised, itchy and now has a non-healing ulcer*

Firm: *yes*

Growing: *yes*

Risk factors

- Unprotected exposure to UV / sunlight over time, during childhood (sunburns): *yes*
- Solarium (tanning bed) use: *none*

Past medical history and family history

- *Hypertension, chronic obstructive pulmonary disease, rheumatoid arthritis*
- *Had a melanoma excised from the back of his wrist 6–7 years ago*
- *Nil family history*

Drug history and allergies

- *Perindopril, amlodipine, Spiriva inhaler, simple analgesics, salbutamol PRN*
- *Long-term low-dose prednisolone for rheumatoid arthritis, Seretide inhaler*
- *NKDA*

Social history

- Smoking history: *30 pack-years*
- Alcohol and drugs history: *3–4 drinks per day, nil illicit drugs*
- *Mobilises with 4-wheel frame*
- *Home with wife who has dementia; patient is full-time carer for her*
- Occupational exposure to UV / sunlight: *worked as a dairy farmer for 40+ years; wore a hat at most times and normal clothing, rarely used sunscreen*

Examination

General inspection (ABCD-V)

- **A**ppearance: *Caucasian man, tanned rough skin*
- **B**ody habitus: *normal, BMI 24*
- **C**ognition: *patient is conscious and oriented*
- **D**evices / **D**rugs: *no*
- **V**itals: *within normal limits*

Complete skin examination

Under normal light and a UVA or black light, the latter of which can help determine whether pigment deposition is epidermal, dermal or mixed:

- Extent of abnormal pigmentation (localised or diffuse) and number of lesions: *abnormal pigmentation localised to one lesion*
- Colour hue: *mixed brown / black colour gradient*
- Morphology of any individual lesions: *crusted ulcer on the left lower border*
- Distribution: *base of neck*
- Pattern: *irregular*
- Closer examination of suspicious individual lesions with a dermatoscope:
  - *8mm asymmetrical lesion with irregular border and appearing raised on base of neck; mixed brown / black colour gradient; crusted ulcer on the left lower border*

Examination of extracutaneous signs as required

- Perform targeted examination
- Cardiovascular: *dual heart sounds, no murmurs*
- Respiratory: *normal breath sounds globally*
- Peripheries: *no evidence of pigmented nail beds (ungual melanoma)*

Investigations

BBMI-O: Bedside, **B**loods, **M**icrobiology, **I**maging and **O**ther

Investigation	Rationale
Bedside	
Bloods	
LDH	Can be useful to support a diagnosis of metastatic melanoma – if elevated, indicates level of tissue damage in other tissues such as liver, brain, lungs

Investigation	Rationale
Microbiology	
Imaging	
▨ CT brain/chest/ abdomen/pelvis	▨ To screen for metastatic spread in stage IV melanoma
Other	
▨ Complete excisional biopsy ▨ Punch/partial incisional/shave biopsy ▨ Sentinel lymph node biopsy	▨ Most optimal biopsy for a suspicious pigmented lesion (complete excision with a 2mm clinical margin and upper subcutis) – melanoma *in situ* is cured by excision because it has no potential to spread around the body ▨ Appropriate in certain clinical situations with experienced clinicians, e.g. large *in situ* lesions, large facial or acral lesions where the suspicion of melanoma is low ▨ Looking for evidence of metastases in malignant lesions

Diagnosis

Melanoma

A patient with a long history of UV exposure, smoking and a new irregular lesion is highly suspicious for melanoma.

The gold standard investigation to confirm melanoma is a complete excisional biopsy.

Discussion

Staging of melanoma helps to determine prognosis, particularly the thickness of the lesion:
▨ Stage 0: <0.1mm thickness
▨ Stage I: <2mm thickness
▨ Stage II: >2mm thickness
▨ Stage III: disease spread to lymph nodes
▨ Stage IV: distant disease spread; usually indicates a poor prognosis

The most common sites for metastases are the liver, lungs, bones and brain.

Management

Lifestyle (preventative)

▨ Surveillance: self-examination, clinical screening by GP/dermatologist, total body photography
▨ Sun exposure reduction and safe sun exposure (wear protective clothes, sunscreen, avoid peak UV times)

Medical

▨ Psychological support and patient education
▨ Radiation: localised radiotherapy, targeted regional node radiation
▨ Chemotherapy (systemic metastases):
  ● Dacarbazine, temozolomide
  ● Immunotherapy: ipilimumab

Surgical

▨ Excision of the lesion: surgical margin of 0.5cm is recommended, wide excision with 1cm margin versus staged excision
▨ Regional lymph node dissection: in metastatic melanoma

Melanoma excision width recommendations

AJCC classification	Breslow thickness	Surgical margin
Stage 0	Melanoma *in situ*	0.5cm
Stage I	Melanoma <1mm	1cm
Stage II	Melanoma 1–4mm	1–2cm
Stage II–III	Melanoma >4mm	2cm

Other differential diagnoses

- Addison's disease (primary adrenal insufficiency)
- Hyperthyroidism
- Diabetic dermopathy
- Acanthosis nigricans
- Hereditary haemochromatosis

Station 59 **Steatorrhoea**

A 40-year-old man presents with a long history of recurrent episodes of epigastric pain.

Tasks

1 Take a history
2 Perform a targeted examination

3 Describe appropriate investigations
4 Formulate a management plan

Differential diagnoses (VIITAMINC)

Vascular

Infective:
- Primary sclerosing cholangitis
- Bacterial overgrowth
- Tropical sprue
- Giardiasis
- Whipple's disease
- HIV / AIDS

Inflammatory:
- Choledocholithiasis
- Primary biliary cirrhosis
- Short gut syndrome
- Inflammatory bowel disease
- Idiopathic pancreatitis

Trauma

Autoimmune

Metabolic:
- Chronic pancreatitis
- Hyperthyroidism

Iatrogenic:
- Resection of stomach, pancreas or small bowel
- Post-cholecystectomy changes
- Medication-related

Neoplastic:
- Lymphoma
- Malignancy

Congenital:
- Coeliac disease
- Zollinger–Ellison syndrome

Other:
- Amyloidosis

Before starting

Establish rapport:
- Introduce yourself
- Obtain consent from the patient: "I'll be asking you questions then performing a physical examination to clarify the cause of your problem. Is this OK with you?"
- Expose the patient: when physical examination is required

Confirm patient details:
- Name   *Allan Hatton*
- Age   *40 years*
- Occupation   *Has found it difficult to find work secondary to recurrent episodes of epigastric pain*

History

History of the presenting complaint

- Severity + quality of the problem:
   - *Foul-smelling stools*
   - *Loose, greasy but bulky-appearing stools*
- Time course:
   - *Occurs episodically*

- Frequency: *results in multiple loose stools each day*
- *Has had a similar event in the past, did not see a doctor*
- Aggravating and relieving factors: *no*
- Associated symptoms:
  - *Persistent unexplained abdominal or gastrointestinal symptoms (i.e. nausea, vomiting, epigastric abdominal pain radiating to the back – particularly worse post a meal, but otherwise fairly constant; the pain is partially relieved by sitting upright or leaning forward); the symptoms last for up to 7 days at a time and have occurred every few months for the past few years*
  - *Unexpected weight loss despite normal eating habits*
    - However, clinically significant protein and fat deficiencies do not occur until >90% of pancreatic function is lost

Past medical history and family history

- *Nil significant past medical history*
- *Nil family history*

Drug history and allergies

- *Antidepressant*
- *NKDA*

Social history

- Smoking history: *15 pack-years*
- Alcohol and drugs history: *up to 10 standard drinks (10 units of alcohol) per day for 5 years secondary to social stressors, only recently been cutting down; nil illicit drugs*

Examination

General inspection (ABCD-V)

- **A**ppearance: *looks uncomfortable on movement*
- **B**ody habitus: *normal, BMI 21*
- **C**ognition: *normal, alert and oriented*
- **D**evices / **D**rugs: *no*
- **V**itals: *BP 130/90mmHg, HR 95bpm, RR 20 per minute; oxygen saturation at 98% on room air; afebrile 37.4°C*

Abdominal examination

- Inspection: *no scars, not distended, no peripheral stigmata of liver disease*
- Palpation: *tender with voluntary guarding in the epigastrium; soft in remainder of abdomen; no hepatosplenomegaly*
- Percussion: *no peritonitis, no ascites*
- Auscultation: *normal bowel sounds*

Investigations

BBMI-O: Bedside, **B**loods, **M**icrobiology, **I**maging and **O**ther

Investigation	Rationale
Bedside	
Bloods	
Serum amylase and lipase	Often normal in patients with chronic pancreatitis (more commonly elevated in acute pancreatitis)
Blood glucose level	
Microbiology	
Stool MCS	Rule out infective cause for loose stools

Investigation	Rationale
Imaging	
▦ Abdominal US	▦ Rule out gallstone disease
▦ CT	▦ Visualise pancreas for any necrosis or pseudocyst formation
▦ MRCP	
▦ Endoscopic US	
Other	
▦ Faecal pancreatic elastase	▦ Looking for severe pancreatic insufficiency

Diagnosis

Chronic pancreatitis

A history of recurrent epigastric pain that radiates to the back associated with steatorrhoea in a patient with chronic alcohol abuse is typical of chronic pancreatitis.

Management

Lifestyle

▦ Chronic alcoholism management (if applicable): reduce / stop alcohol consumption, referral to drug and alcohol specialist units if indicated for counselling and management strategies
▦ Cease smoking
▦ Optimise nutrition and diet: often in conjunction with a dietitian

Medical

▦ Analgesia as required: paracetamol, ibuprofen, tramadol
▦ Antidepressant: indicated for chronic pain management not controlled with analgesia
▦ Pancreatic enzyme replacement therapy (i.e. lipase, pancreatin) in conjunction with a proton pump inhibitor (PPI): in cases of severe malabsorption, can improve steatorrhoea and diarrhoea symptoms; used in conjunction with a PPI to reduce the inactivation of the enzymes by gastric acid

▦ Somatostatin analogue (octreotide)
▦ Parenteral feeding: to minimise the exocrine requirements of the pancreas to induce pancreatic 'resting'

Surgical

▦ Endoscopic retrograde cholangiopancreatography (ERCP) ± pancreatic duct stenting or sphincterotomy
▦ Pancreatic resection: in severe cases where pain and symptoms are not controlled by medical methods:
  ● Pancreaticoduodenectomy
  ● Distal pancreatectomy
▦ Neuroablation: percutaneous radiofrequency ablation of splanchnic nerves for treatment of uncontrolled pain
▦ Extracorporeal shock wave lithotripsy: for pain relief, uncontrolled by medical management

Other differential diagnoses

▦ Coeliac disease

Station 60 **Stoma output**

A 65-year-old woman is 5 days post an emergency Hartmann's procedure (resection of the rectosigmoid colon) for perforated sigmoid diverticulitis. The anorectal stump was closed and a colostomy to redivert faecal material externally was created at the time of operation. On her fluid balance chart, she has been noted to have had an increased stoma output over the past day.

Tasks

1 Take a history
2 Perform a targeted examination
3 Describe appropriate investigations
4 Formulate a management plan

Differential diagnoses (VIITAMINC)

Vascular

Infective:
- Sepsis
- Infection – gastroenteritis, *Clostridium difficile*
- Recurrent diverticulitis in remaining bowel

Inflammatory:
- Dysmotility disorders

Trauma

Autoimmune

Metabolic

Iatrogenic:
- Post bowel resection
- Subacute obstruction
- Radiation enteritis
- Medication-related – steroid withdrawal, prokinetic agents, laxatives

Neoplastic

Congenital

Other

Before starting

Establish rapport:
- Introduce yourself
- Obtain consent from the patient: "I will be asking you some questions and then will be performing a physical examination to find out why you have a problem with your stoma output. Is this OK with you?"
- Expose the patient: when physical examination is required

Confirm patient details:
- Name — *Annie Smart*
- Age — *65 years*
- Occupation — *Retired*

History

Exposures
- Recent travel: *none*
- Change in diet: *none*
- Sick contacts: *none; however a patient in a neighbouring cubicle had diarrhoea contact precautions*
- Medication-related: *the patient had antibiotics administered during her hospital admission*

Associated symptoms
- *Loose, watery stoma output*
- *Some dry mouth / thirst, fatigue and abdominal cramps*

- *Abdominal pain, bloating, nausea, vomiting, lack of flatus for 18 hours*
- Fever / rigors, malaise and general unwellness: *patient states feeling generally unwell lately, no fevers or rigors*

Examination

General inspection (ABCD-V)

- **A**ppearance: *looks unwell*
- **B**ody habitus: *normal, BMI 24*
- **C**ognition: *normal, alert and oriented*
- **D**evices / **D**rugs: *the indwelling catheter is draining concentrated tea-coloured urine, IV fluids are running at a 12-hourly rate*
- **V**itals: *BP 100/60mmHg, HR 110bpm, RR 21 per minute; oxygen saturation at 97% on room air; low-grade temperature 37.9°C*

Fluid review

- Check perfusion of peripheries (*normal*), tissue turgor (*slow*)
- Check jugular venous pressure (*not elevated*), mucous membranes (*dry*)

- Listen to heart and chest: *heart sounds dual, nil added; chest is clear*
- *No evidence of peripheral and sacral oedema*
- Review of fluid balance charts (fluid input and output): *negative balance over past day secondary to high stoma output*

Abdominal examination

- Inspection: *midline laparotomy scar is dressed; the dressing appears dry and intact; a stoma is sited on the left lower abdomen*
- Palpation: *examine for distension and tenderness on palpation*
- Percussion: *no percussive tenderness or peritonitis; no ascites*
- Auscultation: *bowel sounds are overactive*
- With assistance (from the patient or nursing staff), the stoma bag can be taken down and the stoma inspected; look at the appearance of the mucosa, note its activity and its output contents: *the stoma contents are a very watery brown colour; the stoma itself appears healthy*

Investigations

BBMI-O: Bedside, **B**loods, **M**icrobiology, **I**maging and **O**ther

Investigation	Rationale
Bedside	
ECG	For patients with hypokalaemia
Bloods	
FBC	Looking for signs of infection
U&Es and creatinine, CMP	Assessing renal function, electrolytes
CRP	Looking for signs of infection
Microbiology	
Stool MCS + *C. difficile* toxin	Rule out a gastrointestinal infective cause; testing for other infective causes in stool such as specific parasites could be appropriate if the history indicates these exposures

Investigation	Rationale
Imaging	
▦ AXR + CT abdomen	▦ Imaging for obstruction, pseudo-obstruction, dilatation / thickening of the bowel, inflammatory change secondary to infection, other sources of intra-abdominal sepsis
Other	

Diagnosis

C. difficile colitis

An acute increase in stomal output on the background of recent antibiotic use must be thoroughly investigated for *C. difficile*.

The gold standard investigation to confirm C. difficile *colitis is stool MCS with* C. difficile *toxin.*

Discussion

Pseudomembranous colitis due to *C. difficile* toxin commonly occurs after recent broad-spectrum antibiotic therapy (e.g. cephalosporins) due to disruption of the normal bowel flora.

High output stoma: >2000ml/day for >3 days or 1000–2000ml/day if <200cm small bowel remaining or ongoing hydration / electrolyte abnormalities.

Stomas can be created temporarily or permanently for the management of a variety of conditions, including congenital anomalies, large bowel obstruction, inflammatory bowel disease, intestinal trauma or gastrointestinal malignancy.

Anatomic location and type of stoma constructed have an impact on management. The type and volume of output, and therefore fluid loss, are determined by the location of the stoma relative to the ileocaecal valve. Contents by the end of the ileum thus can be expected to have more of a fluid consistency, whereas that from the colon can be expected to have more of a solid consistency.

Intestinal stomas include the ileostomy and the colostomy:

▦ An **ileostomy** is when the open end of the ileum (small intestine) is brought to the surface of the abdomen and secured there to form an exit for bowel contents; ileostomies are most often sited on the right side of the abdomen; ileostomy fluid is alkaline and rich in proteolytic enzymes; as the contents are more irritating to the skin, they are 'spouted' (or protruding) out from the abdominal wall so that the faecal content can drain into the stoma bag without contacting the skin.

• Average ileostomy output ranges from 500ml/day to 1300ml/day

• In the early postoperative period and in episodes of gastroenteritis this can increase to 1800ml/day or even higher

• The ileostomy fluid contains high amounts of sodium and potassium

▦ A **colostomy** (permanent or temporary) is when the open end of the colon (large intestine) is brought to the surface of the abdomen and secured there to form an exit for faecal matter. Colostomies are most often sited on the left side of the abdomen, and are often 'flush' to the skin (i.e. not protruding outwards like an ileostomy) because their contents are less irritating to the skin.

Management

Medical

- Discontinue causative agent (if still taking)
- Analgesia as required
- Anti-emetics if indicated
- IV fluid rehydration: bolus for loss and ongoing maintenance

- Metronidazole: first-line, 10-day course
- Vancomycin (oral): in severe disease, 10-day course
- Faecal microbiota transplantation: in cases of recurrent episodes where other medical managements have failed

Surgical

- Bowel resection (colectomy): in severe cases, especially if severe organ dysfunction or toxic megacolon development

Other differential diagnoses

- Post bowel resection

Station 61 **Stridor**

A 70-year-old man presents with a 24-hour history of stridor.

Tasks

1 Take a history
2 Perform a targeted examination
3 Describe appropriate investigations
4 Formulate a management plan

Differential diagnoses (VIITAMINC)

Vascular:
- Subglottic haemangioma
- Stroke

Infective:
- Laryngitis
- Epiglottitis / supraglottitis
- Tracheitis
- Deep neck space infection

Inflammatory:
- Laryngopharyngeal reflux

Trauma:
- Laryngeal fracture
- Glottic web

Autoimmune:
- Connective tissue disorders (systemic lupus erythematosus / rheumatoid arthritis)

Metabolic:
- Hypokalaemia
- Anaphylaxis

Iatrogenic / idiopathic:
- Vocal cord granuloma (secondary to intubation)
- Subglottic stenosis
- Paradoxical vocal cord movement
- Iatrogenic recurrent laryngeal nerve palsy (post surgical, prolonged intubation, etc.)
- Foreign body

Neoplastic / neurological:
- Laryngeal malignancy
- Recurrent respiratory papillomatosis

Congenital:
- Laryngomalacia

Before starting

Establish rapport:
- Introduce yourself
- Obtain consent from the patient: "I'll be asking you questions, then performing a physical examination to find out why you have noisy breathing. Is this OK with you?"
- Expose the patient: when physical examination is required

Confirm patient details:
- Name — *Mark Hemmings*
- Age — *70 years*
- Occupation — *Retired carpenter*

History

History of presenting complaint

- History of stridor:
  - *Ongoing for the past 24 hours*
  - *On the background of 2 days of cough and runny nose*
- Quality of stridor:
  - *Biphasic stridor*
  - *Present at rest*
  - *Worsened with exertion*
- Associated symptoms:
  - *Shortness of breath*
  - *Associated neck pain*

- *Odynophagia and dysphagia*
- *Nil recent weight loss, night sweats or other systemic symptoms*

Past medical history and family history

- *Gastro-oesophageal reflux disease, ischaemic heart disease*
- *Mother had bowel cancer*

Drug history and allergies

- *Perindopril*
- *NKDA*

Social history

- Smoking history: *25 pack-years*
- Alcohol and drugs history: *social drinker, nil illicit drugs*

Examination

General inspection (ABCD-V)

- **A**ppearance: *significant respiratory distress with accessory muscle use; unable to speak in full sentences*
- **B**ody habitus: *overweight, BMI 29*
- **C**ognition: *patient is conscious and oriented*
- **D**evices/**D**rugs: *nil*
- **V**itals: *BP 120/70mmHg, HR 100bpm, RR 27 per minute; oxygen saturation at 98% on room air; afebrile*

Head and neck examination

- Inspection: *obvious biphasic stridor at rest; otherwise no surgical scars, deformities, obvious goitre, other masses or obvious craniofacial deformities*
- Palpation: *generalised tenderness in neck, worse over the larynx; bilateral cervical lymphadenopathy; no palpable goitre; no other palpable masses*

ENT examination

- Ear:
  - Otoscopy: *nothing abnormal detected*
  - Weber and Rinne: *nothing abnormal detected*
- Nose: *nothing abnormal detected*
- Throat: *mild erythema of posterior pharyngeal wall, no oedema*

Flexible nasoendoscopy / mirror laryngoscopy

- Nasopharynx/oropharynx: *nothing abnormal detected*
- Larynx/hypopharynx: *significantly erythematous and oedematous supraglottic structures; 70% obstruction of vocal cords*
- Subglottis: *nothing abnormal detected*

Neurological examination

- *All assessable cranial nerves intact*
- *Upper and lower limb tone, power, reflexes, sensation and coordination all intact*

Investigations

BBMI-O: Bedside, **B**loods, **M**icrobiology, **I**maging and **O**ther

Investigation	Rationale
Bedside	
Bloods	
FBC	Looking for raised white cell count
CRP	Looking for infection
U&Es and creatinine	Looking for renal impairment / electrolyte abnormality

Investigation	Rationale
Microbiology	
Imaging	
▦ CT head and neck	▦ Consider if diagnosis still unclear
Other	

Diagnosis

Supraglottitis

A patient with recent upper respiratory tract infection symptoms that now presents with erythematous and oedematous supraglottic structures with 70% obstruction is concerning for supraglottitis.

Management

The first and most important step in managing a patient with compromised airway is to ensure a secured airway. DO NOT delay in securing the airway to obtain imaging / bloods / other investigations, etc.

Management of airway

- ▦ Medical:
  - ● Assess safety of airway – if there are any concerns call for help from an experienced physician
  - ● Consider the need for immediate intubation to secure the airway
  - ● Consider the need for HDU or high visual bed monitoring
- ▦ Surgical management of airway:
  - ● Needle cricothyroidotomy
  - ● Surgical cricothyroidotomy
  - ● Surgical tracheostomy

Management of supraglottitis

- ▦ Nebulised adrenaline
- ▦ High-dose corticosteroid (usually dexamethasone)
- ▦ Broad-spectrum antibiotics (flucloxacillin, ceftriaxone, metronidazole)

Other differential diagnoses

- ▦ Deep neck space infection
- ▦ Tracheitis
- ▦ Glottic web
- ▦ Vocal cord granuloma
- ▦ Subglottic stenosis
- ▦ Foreign body
- ▦ Recurrent respiratory papillomatosis
- ▦ Laryngomalacia

Station 62 **Syncope**

An 81-year-old man has been brought in to the emergency department by ambulance with an unwitnessed syncopal episode at home.

Tasks

1 Take a history
2 Perform a targeted examination

3 Describe appropriate investigations
4 Formulate a management plan

Differential diagnoses (VIITAMINC)

Vascular:
- Acute myocardial infarction (AMI)
- Valvular heart disease
- Dehydration
- Anaemia
- Arrhythmia
- Aortic dissection
- Pulmonary embolism
- Cerebrovascular accident (CVA) / transient ischaemic attack (TIA)
- Intracranial haemorrhage

Infective / **I**nflammatory:
- Sepsis

Trauma:
- Head trauma
- Haemorrhage

Autoimmune:
- Connective tissue disorders (systemic lupus erythematosus / rheumatoid arthritis)

Metabolic:
- Anaphylaxis
- Hypoglycaemia / hyperglycaemia
- Uraemia / hepatic encephalopathy

Iatrogenic / **I**diopathic:
- Pseudoseizures
- Vasovagal syncope
- Drugs / intoxication

Neoplastic:
- Atrial myxoma

Congenital:
- Cardiomyopathy
- Epilepsy
- Orthostatic hypotension

Before starting

Establish rapport:
- Introduce yourself
- Obtain consent from the patient: "I'll be asking you questions then perform a physical exam to find out why you collapsed. Is this OK with you?"
- Expose the patient: when physical examination is required

Confirm patient details:
- Name — *James Field*
- Age — *81 years*
- Occupation — *Retired engineer*

History

History of presenting complaint

- History of syncope: *unwitnessed, stood up from chair, 20 seconds of palpitations / racing heart and feeling faint, next thing he remembers*

is waking up on the floor, unsure of duration;
unable to get up off the floor so called the
ambulance
- Associated symptoms:
  - Recent mild viral gastroenteritis with some
    nausea and diarrhoea over the past 4 days
  - Mildly disoriented/confused
  - Denies aura
  - Denies chest pain/shortness of breath
  - Denies all else

Past medical history and family history

- Type 2 diabetes mellitus, hypertension,
  hypercholesterolaemia, atrial fibrillation, chronic
  kidney disease, chronic back pain, gastro-
  oesophageal reflux disease, chronic obstructive
  pulmonary disease
- Nil family history

Drug history and allergies

- Perindopril, NovoMix 30, metformin XR, gliclazide,
  rosuvastatin, warfarin, pregabalin, Seretide,
  Ventolin MDI PRN, pantoprazole
- NKDA

Social history

- Smoking history: 40 pack-years
- Alcohol and drugs history: non-drinker, used to
  drink 4–5 standard units per week for 10 years;
  nil illicit drugs
- Lives home alone – home help three times per
  week
- Mobilises with single point stick

Examination

General inspection (ABCD-V)

- **A**ppearance: frail elderly man
- **B**ody habitus: normal, BMI 20
- **C**ognition: Glasgow Coma Scale (GCS) 14,
  disoriented and confused

- **D**evices/**D**rugs: nil
- **V**itals: BP 90/70mmHg, HR 100bpm irregular,
  RR 27 per minute; oxygen saturation at 98% on
  room air; temperature 37.4°C

Neurological examination

- Poorly compliant with examination due to
  confusion; however, cranial nerves grossly intact
  and upper and lower limbs grossly neurologically
  intact

Cardiovascular examination

- Inspection:
  - No obvious chest wall deformities/scars,
    no presence of a pacemaker
  - No palmar pallor or conjunctival pallor
  - Jugular venous pressure 0cm (at sternal notch)
  - Dry mucous membranes
  - No peripheral oedema
- Palpation:
  - Pulses (radial) strong, irregularly irregular
    rhythm
  - No palpable thrill or heave
  - No pitting oedema peripherally
- Auscultation:
  - Dual heart sounds
  - Irregularly irregular rhythm
  - No murmurs heard, no added heart sounds

Respiratory examination

- Normal vesicular breath sounds throughout
- Nil added sounds

Abdominal examination

- Abdomen soft and non-tender
- Nil palpable organomegaly

Secondary survey

- Abrasion to left shoulder and upper arm; mild
  tenderness to palpation; no obvious deformity
- No traumatic head injury; no cervical spine
  tenderness

Investigations

BBMI-O: Bedside, **B**loods, **M**icrobiology, **I**maging and **O**ther

Investigations	Rationale
Bedside	
ECG	Investigate for AMI / arrhythmias
Postural BPs	Investigate for orthostatic hypotension
Mini mental state examination / cognitive screen	Assess the likelihood of underlying dementia
Bloods	
FBC	Looking for raised WCC or low Hb
CRP	Looking for infection
U&Es and creatinine	Looking for renal impairment / electrolyte abnormality
CMP	Looking for electrolyte abnormality
Coagulation studies	Looking for raised INR
LFTs	Looking for acutely deranged liver function
Troponin	Looking for evidence of AMI
Blood sugar level + ketones	Looking for hypo- / hyperglycaemia
Ammonia	Consider hepatic encephalopathy in deranged LFTs and new confusion
Microbiology	
Imaging	
CT brain	Investigate for CVA and spontaneous or traumatic intracranial haemorrhage, given unwitnessed fall on warfarin
CXR	Investigate for acute pulmonary oedema, cardiomegaly, consolidation
Left shoulder and humerus XR	Investigate for fractures
Other	
24-hour Holter / ECG monitoring	Consider if arrhythmia likely or no other cause found
Echocardiogram	Consider if investigating valvular heart disease, atrial myxoma, etc.

Diagnosis

Orthostatic syncopal episode in the setting of viral gastroenteritis and subsequent dehydration

This patient is clinically dehydrated, likely on the background of his gastroenteritis, and has given a history that is consistent with postural syncope.

Other differential diagnoses

- Acute coronary syndrome
- Valvular heart disease
- Arrhythmia
- Anaemia
- Sepsis
- Head trauma / intracranial haemorrhage
- Hypoglycaemia
- Vasovagal syncope
- Stroke / TIA
- Cardiomyopathy

Station 63 **Testicular mass**

A 35-year-old man presents to the GP with a 2-month history of a scrotal lump.

Tasks

1 Take a history
2 Perform a targeted examination

3 Describe appropriate investigations
4 Formulate a management plan

Differential diagnosis (VIITAMINC)

Vascular

Infective:
- Epididymo-orchitis

Inflammatory:
- Hydrocele
- Varicocele

Trauma:
- Testicular torsion
- Torsion of the testicular appendage

Autoimmune

Metabolic

Iatrogenic

Neoplastic:
- Testicular carcinoma

Congenital:
- Inguinal hernia

Other

Before starting

Establish rapport:
- Introduce yourself
- Obtain consent from the patient: "I'll be asking you questions, and then performing a physical exam. Is this OK with you?"
- Expose the patient: when physical examination is required inform the patient that the area you will examine is exposed appropriately

Confirm patient details:
- Name   *Joseph Lightfoot*
- Age   *35 years*
- Occupation   *Bricklayer*

History

History of presenting complaint

- History of scrotal mass: *left-sided 1cm lump, 2 months, slowly enlarging, not painful*
- Associated symptoms: *no loss of weight, no fevers/chills/rigors, no history of trauma,*

no genitourinary symptoms, no back pain, no chest pain

Past medical history and family history

- *Chronic bronchitis, gastro-oesophageal reflux disease*
- *Father had testicular cancer at age 27 years*

Drug history and allergies

- *Pantoprazole*
- *Ventolin MDI PRN*
- *NKDA*

Social history

- Smoking history: *15 pack-years*
- Alcohol and drugs history: *social drinker, nil illicit drugs*
- *Lives at home with wife and three children*

Examination

General inspection (ABCD-V)

- **A**ppearance: *fit and healthy young man*
- **B**ody habitus: *normal, BMI 22*

- **C**ognition: *patient is conscious and oriented*
- **D**evices / **D**rugs: *nil*
- **V**itals: *BP 120/70mmHg, HR 70bpm, RR 27/min; oxygen saturation at 98% on room air; afebrile*

Genital examination

- Inspection: *no skin changes, no obvious lump visible; does not transilluminate; no blue dot sign (testicular appendage torsion)*
- Palpation: *left-sided 1cm lump separate from testes, unable to palpate above lump; the lump is soft and non-tender, able to be reduced into inguinal canal; cough impulse palpable; no inguinal lymphadenopathy; no testicular masses*
- *Cremasteric reflex intact*

Investigations

BBMI-O: Bedside, **B**loods, **M**icrobiology, **I**maging and **O**ther

Investigations	Rationale
Bedside	
Bloods	
FBC	Looking for raised WCC
CRP	Looking for infection
U&Es and creatinine	Looking for renal impairment / electrolyte abnormality
Alpha-fetoprotein	Consider in testicular cancer
HCG	Consider in testicular cancer
LDH	Consider in testicular cancer
Microbiology	
Urine MCS	Consider in epididymitis / orchitis
Imaging	
US inguinal / scrotum	First-line investigation in all inguinal / scrotal masses
CT pelvis	Looking for pelvic / abdominal masses
Other	

Diagnosis

Inguinal hernia

Despite a family history of testicular cancer, the examination is clinically suggestive of an inguinal hernia.

The gold standard investigation to confirm an inguinal hernia is via history and examination or inguinal US.

Management

Adjunct

- Supportive underwear
- Treat chronic coughing / straining and avoid postoperatively for up to 6 weeks
- Monitor for recurrence or contralateral occurrence
- Monitor for postoperative complications (haematomas, seroma, wound infection, chronic pain)

Medical

- Up to a third of patients with inguinal hernias will never experience any symptoms
- Conservative management can be considered in these patients, with the education that future surgical intervention is likely and information regarding the signs and symptoms of complication (i.e. strangulation, incarceration)

Surgical

- Surgical inguinal hernia repair (open, laparoscopic)

Other differential diagnoses

- Testicular torsion
- Torsion of testicular appendage
- Epididymo-orchitis
- Testicular carcinoma
- Hydrocele
- Varicocele
- Spermatocele

Station 64 **Tremor**

An 85-year-old woman presents to the GP with a 6-month history of worsening tremor.

Tasks

1 Take a history
2 Perform a targeted examination
3 Describe appropriate investigations
4 Formulate a management plan

Differential diagnosis (VIITAMINC)

Vascular:
- Stroke

Infective

Inflammatory

Trauma

Autoimmune:
- Multiple sclerosis

Metabolic:
- Physiological tremor
- Hypoglycaemia
- Hyperthyroidism

Iatrogenic:
- Medication-induced tremor

Neoplastic:
- Intracranial tumour

Congenital:
- Wilson's disease

Other:
- Parkinson's disease
- Essential tremor
- Psychogenic tremor

Before starting

Establish rapport:
- Introduce yourself
- Obtain consent from the patient: "I'll be asking you questions, and then performing a physical examination to find out why you have tremor. Is this OK with you?"
- Expose the patient: when physical examination is required

Confirm patient details:
- Name — *Mary Heal*
- Age — *85 years*
- Occupation — *Retired pharmacist*

History

History of presenting complaint

- History of tremor: *past 6 months, insidious onset, slowly worsening, confined to hands*
- Quality of tremor: *worse at rest; tremor is reduced or disappears entirely when movement is initiated; left hand worse than right*
- Associated symptoms: *some new memory issues recently, no stimulant intake, no symptoms of stroke / transient ischaemic attack, no symptoms of hypo- / hyperthyroidism*

Past medical history and family history

- *Type 2 diabetes mellitus, hypertension, hypercholesterolaemia, ischaemic heart disease, chronic kidney disease, diverticular disease, depression*

▨ *Mother had bowel cancer, father had dementia, brother has dementia*

Drug history and allergies

▨ *Metformin, gliclazide, ramipril, atorvastatin, aspirin, metoprolol, venlafaxine*

▨ *NKDA*

Social history

▨ Smoking history: *20 pack-years*

▨ Alcohol and drugs history: *social drinker, nil illicit drugs*

▨ *Lives at home alone*

Examination

General inspection (ABCD-V)

▨ **A**ppearance: *stuttering speech, shuffling gait, obvious low-frequency pill-rolling left hand tremor at rest, slight mask facies*

▨ **B**ody habitus: *overweight, BMI 29*

▨ **C**ognition: *patient is alert and oriented, loses track of conversation occasionally*

▨ **D**evices/**D**rugs: *nil*

▨ **V**itals: *BP 120/70mmHg no postural drop, HR 80bpm, RR 27 per minute; oxygen saturation at 98% on room air; afebrile*

Neurological examination

▨ Upper limb: *cogwheel rigidity, global 4+/5 weakness, hyperreflexia, slight dysdiadochokinesis, slight past-pointing*

▨ Lower limb: *cogwheel rigidity, 5/5 power, hyperreflexia with sustained clonus, slight incoordination*

▨ Cranial nerves: *all intact*

▨ Parkinson's examination: *positive glabellar tap, micrographia, festinating speech*

Thyroid examination

▨ Inspection:
  ● *No goitre*
  ● *No proptosis*
  ● *No pretibial myxoedema*
  ● *No proximal muscle wasting*

▨ Palpation: *no palpable thyroid lumps*

▨ Percussion: *no retrosternal dullness*

▨ Auscultation: *no thyroid bruits*

Investigations

BBMI-O: Bedside, **B**loods, **M**icrobiology, **I**maging and **O**ther

Investigation	Rationale
Bedside	
Bloods	
▨ U&Es and creatinine	▨ Looking for renal impairment/electrolyte abnormality
▨ TFTs	▨ Looking for thyroid dysfunction
▨ Serum copper and caeruloplasmin	▨ Looking for Wilson's disease
▨ Serum glucose	▨ Looking for hypo-/hyperglycaemia
Microbiology	

Investigation	Rationale
Imaging	
CT brain	If considering cerebrovascular accident or brainstem / cerebellar tumour
MRI brain + spine	Looking for demyelination plaques if considering multiple sclerosis
Renal US	Good first-line investigation in renal function abnormality
Thyroid US	Good first-line investigation in thyroid function abnormality
Other	

Diagnosis

Parkinson's disease

This patient presents with many symptoms of Parkinson's disease, such as a pill-rolling tremor, a shuffling gait and cogwheel rigidity.

Management

Medical

- Levodopa + carbidopa / benserazide (e.g. Madopar, Sinemet)
- Dopamine agonist (e.g. bromocriptine, pramipexole)
- Glutamate antagonist (amantadine)
- Catechol-O-methyltransferase (COMT) inhibitor (entacapone):
  - Monoamine oxidase B (MAO-B) inhibitor (selegiline, rasagiline)

Psychological and psychiatric

- Antidepressants
- Antidementia agents (rivastigmine, donepezil)
- Antipsychotics (quetiapine – lowest rate of extrapyramidal side-effects)
- Cognitive behavioural therapy (CBT) for impulsive behaviours
- Benzodiazepines for sleep

Adjuncts

- Speech and swallow therapy
- Exercise therapy

Surgical

- Deep brain stimulation

Other differential diagnoses

- Essential tremor
- Physiological tremor
- Medication-induced tremor
- Multiple sclerosis
- Cerebellar or brainstem tumour
- Stroke
- Psychogenic tremor

Station 65 **Vision changes**

A 35-year-old man presents to his GP with a 1-hour history of visual changes.

Tasks

1 Take a history
2 Perform a targeted examination

3 Describe appropriate investigations
4 Formulate a management plan

Differential diagnoses (VIITAMINC)

Vascular:
- Retinal artery occlusion
- Retinal vein occlusion
- Postural hypotension
- Vertebrobasilar stroke

Infective:
- Endophthalmitis

Inflammatory:
- Episcleritis
- Acute angle closure glaucoma

Trauma:
- Intraocular foreign body
- Corneal ulcer
- Retinal detachment

Autoimmune:
- Giant cell arteritis
- Optic neuritis

Metabolic:
- Vitreous haemorrhage

Iatrogenic/**I**diopathic

Neoplastic/**N**eurological:
- Orbital tumour

Congenital

Other:
- Ocular migraine

Before starting

Establish rapport:
- Introduce yourself
- Obtain consent from the patient: "I'll be asking you questions, and then performing a physical examination to find out why your vision has changed. Is this OK with you?"
- Expose the patient: when physical examination is required

Confirm patient details:
- Name   *Bartosz Kwjatkovski*
- Age   *35 years*
- Occupation   *Construction worker*

History

History of presenting complaint

- History of visual loss: *at home, flashing lights and zig-zag lines for a few minutes before vision deteriorated, complete visual loss over the course of minutes; only left eye affected, never happened before*
- Associated symptoms: *associated nausea and vomiting, denies headache, denies orbital pain, denies presyncopal episode, denies jaw claudication, shoulder pain, denies all other symptoms*

Past medical history and family history

- Classical migraines, type 2 diabetes mellitus, hypertension
- Mother has Graves' disease

Drug history and allergies

- Perindopril, metformin, sumatriptan PRN
- NKDA

Social history

- Smoking history: 30 pack-years
- Alcohol and drugs history: non-drinker, nil illicit drugs

Examination

General inspection (ABCD-V)

- **A**ppearance: distressed
- **B**ody habitus: obese, BMI 33
- **C**ognition: patient is conscious and oriented
- **D**evices / **D**rugs: nil
- **V**itals: BP 140/80mmHg, HR 90bpm, RR 20 per minute; oxygen saturation at 99% on room air; afebrile

Eye examination

- Inspection: no ptosis, proptosis, injection or chemosis
- Visual acuity: right eye 6/6, left eye hand motion only; not corrected with pinhole
- Visual fields: right eye normal, left eye unable to assess
- Pupil assessment: pupils equal and reactive to light; no relative afferent pupillary defect (RAPD)
- Colour vision: no red desaturation; Ishihara colour testing – nothing abnormal detected
- Fluorescein stain and slit lamp: no corneal abrasions; no other abnormalities

Cranial nerves

- Optic nerve examination as above
- CN III, IV, VI: no ophthalmoplegia
- All other cranial nerves intact

Neurological examination

- Upper and lower limb tone, power, reflexes, sensation and coordination all intact

Diabetic examination

- No microvascular, macrovascular or autonomic complications

Investigations

BBMI-O: Bedside, **B**loods, **M**icrobiology, **I**maging and **O**ther

Investigation	Rationale
Bedside	
ECG	Investigate for arrhythmias
Bloods	
FBC	Looking for raised WCC and thrombocytosis
U&Es and creatinine	Looking for renal function in diabetes
CRP	Looking for inflammation
ESR	Looking for inflammation
Coagulation studies	Looking for bleeding diathesis
Thrombophilia screen	Looking for thrombophilia
Microbiology	

Investigation	Rationale
Imaging	
Carotid Doppler or angiography	If considering vertebrobasilar stroke
Fluorescein angiography	To investigate for retinal vascular occlusion
CT brain / MRI with perfusion studies	To investigate for stroke, multiple sclerosis plaques
Other	
Fundoscopy	Essential in all episodes of visual loss
Echocardiogram (transthoracic echo)	Investigate source for potential thromboemboli
Temporal artery biopsy	If investigating giant cell arteritis
Tonometry	If considering acute angle closure glaucoma

Diagnosis

Ocular migraine

In a previously well patient with a history of classical migraines, it is not uncommon for ocular phenomena to arise.

Management

Ocular migraines are generally benign and self-limiting, with most episodes only lasting up to 30–40 minutes.

Non-medical management

- Reassurance
- Avoiding trigger foods (chocolate, caffeine, spicy foods, etc.)
- Adequate sleep hygiene
- Avoid stress
- Biofeedback or cognitive behavioural therapy (CBT)

Medical management

- Analgesia: NSAIDs, opioids
- Abortive medications: ergotamine, triptans
- Anti-emetics
- Preventative medications: anti-epileptics, antidepressants, antihypertensives
- Transcranial magnetic stimulation

Other differential diagnoses

- Postural hypotension
- Endophthalmitis
- Foreign body
- Corneal ulcer
- Retinal detachment

Station 66 **Voice changes**

A 50-year-old woman presents to the GP with a 3-month history of voice changes.

Tasks

1 Take a history
2 Perform a targeted examination
3 Describe appropriate investigations
4 Formulate a management plan

Differential diagnoses (VIITAMINC)

Vascular:
- Haemangioma
- Stroke

Infective:
- Laryngitis
- Epiglottitis

Inflammatory:
- Laryngopharyngeal reflux
- Reinke's oedema (smoking)

Trauma:
- Voice abuse
- Laryngeal fracture
- Arytenoid dislocation
- Chemical inhalational injuries
- Intubation
- Presbylaryngis

Autoimmune:
- Connective tissue disorders (systemic lupus erythematosus / rheumatoid arthritis)

Metabolic:
- Hypothyroidism

Iatrogenic

Neoplastic:
- Laryngeal cancers
- Laryngeal nodules / cysts

Congenital:
- Congenital laryngeal web

Other:
- Psychogenic
- Functional dysphonia
- Vocal fold paralysis

Before starting

Establish rapport:
- Introduce yourself
- Obtain consent from the patient: "I'll be asking you questions, and then performing a physical examination to find out why you have voice changes. Is this OK with you?"
- Expose the patient: when physical examination is required

Confirm patient details:
- Name   *Sonia Wood*
- Age   *60 years*
- Occupation   *Teacher*

History

History of presenting complaint

- History of dysphonia: *past 3 months, constant, onset after upper respiratory tract infection 3 months ago, slowly worsening, worse at end of the day, affecting ability to work*
- Quality of dysphonia: *harshness / huskiness to voice, normal projection, no breathiness, no increased work*
- Associated symptoms: *occasional reflux, no dysphagia, no odynophagia, no weight loss, no other systemic symptoms*

Past medical history and family history

- Gastro-oesophageal reflux disease, ischaemic heart disease
- Mother had hypothyroidism

Drug history and allergies

- Perindopril, omeprazole
- NKDA

Social history

- Smoking history: 30 pack-years
- Alcohol and drugs history: social drinker, nil illicit drugs

Examination

General inspection (ABCD-V)

- **A**ppearance: dressed appropriately, not cachectic; no respiratory distress/accessory muscle use; no noisy breathing
- **B**ody habitus: overweight, BMI 27
- **C**ognition: patient is conscious and oriented
- **D**evices/**D**rugs: nil
- **V**itals: BP 120/70mmHg, HR 70bpm, RR 18 per minute; oxygen saturation at 98% on room air; afebrile

Head and neck examination

- Inspection: no surgical scars, deformities, obvious goitre, other masses or obvious craniofacial deformities
- Palpation: 2 × 3cm nodular mass felt in upper left neck; fixed immobile, rubbery, mildly tender; no overlying skin changes; does not move on swallowing or sticking out tongue; no palpable goitre; no other palpable masses

- Percussion: no retrosternal expansion of thyroid lobe
- Auscultation: no audible bruits heard over the thyroid gland

ENT examination

- Ear:
  - Otoscopy: nothing abnormal detected
  - Weber and Rinne tests: nothing abnormal detected
- Nose: no engorged turbinates, septal deviation or obstruction noted
- Throat: no oral abnormalities seen, no soft palate swelling, uvula midline, no masses/lesions in oral cavity or oropharynx

Flexible nasoendoscopy/mirror laryngoscopy

- Nasopharynx/oropharynx: no obvious abnormalities
- Laryngeal vestibule: no obvious abnormalities; epiglottis normal; aryepiglottic folds normal, piriform sinuses normal; false vocal folds normal; no oedema
- Glottis: large nodular mass in the anterior left true vocal fold invading into thyroid lamina, no other masses seen; bilateral vocal fold movement with apposition of vocal folds; mass not concerning for airway compromise yet
- Subglottis: no obvious abnormality

Neurological examination

- All assessable cranial nerves intact
- Upper and lower limb tone, power, reflexes, sensation and coordination all intact

Investigations

BBMI-O: **B**edside, **B**loods, **M**icrobiology, **I**maging and **O**ther

Investigation	Rationale
Bedside	
▨ ECG	▨ Preoperative to assess fitness for surgery
Bloods	
▨ FBC	▨ Looking for anaemia
▨ U&Es and creatinine	▨ Looking for renal impairment / electrolyte abnormality
▨ TFTs	▨ Looking for hyper- / hypothyroidism
Microbiology	
Imaging	
▨ CT head and neck	▨ Looking for laryngeal malignancy
▨ MRI head and neck	▨ Further characterisation of laryngeal mass
▨ US neck / thyroid ± FNA	▨ Help to differentiate thyroid node / cyst versus lymph node
▨ Consider staging CT CAP	▨ To look for metastases (depending on TNM staging of primary)
▨ Consider fused PET / CT	▨ If location / nodal involvement is unclear
▨ Consider Tc-99m thyroid scan	▨ If primary thyroid nodule to assess function
Other	
▨ Pulmonary function tests	▨ Given past history of smoking, to assess fitness for surgery
▨ Echo	▨ Given past history of ischaemic heart disease, to assess fitness for surgery

---

Diagnosis

Glottic squamous cell carcinoma with clinically involved neck lymph node

While difficult to distinguish the lymph node from a thyroid nodule, the findings from endoscopy show a glottic mass that, in an older patient with a long smoking history, is very suspicious for malignancy.

Pan-endoscopy + biopsy are necessary for diagnosis of laryngeal cancer.

Management

Medical

- Ensure airway not threatened by glottic mass
- Consider admission with early referral to ICU if threatened airway
- Obtain functional studies to assess fitness for surgery as above

Surgical management of primary tumour

- Depending on location and size of tumour
- Surgical management of the primary tumour may involve primary radiotherapy ± cordectomy all the way through to total laryngectomy with postoperative chemoradiotherapy for advanced tumours

Surgical management of neck node

- Elective neck dissections are NOT clinically indicated (i.e. when there are no clinically palpable lymph nodes)
- When clinical lymph nodes are present, primary radiotherapy, modified radical or selective neck dissection may be indicated depending on the tumour staging

Other differential diagnoses

- Haemangioma
- Laryngitis
- Reinke's oedema
- Laryngopharyngeal reflux
- Voice abuse
- Laryngeal nodules / cyst

Station 67 **Vomiting**

A 35-year-old woman presents to the emergency department with a 1-day history of vomiting and abdominal pain.

Tasks

1 Take history
2 Perform physical examination

3 Provide rationale for investigations
4 Formulate a management plan

Differential diagnoses (VIITAMINC)

Vascular

Infective:
- Food poisoning
- Viral gastroenteritis
- Urinary tract infection (UTI)/pyelonephritis

Inflammatory:
- Vestibular dysfunction (labyrinthitis, benign paroxysmal positional vertigo)
- Raised intracranial pressure
- Acute abdomen
- Obstruction (small/large bowel obstruction, achalasia, pyloric stenosis)
- Renal calculi
- Ovarian torsion

Trauma

Autoimmune

Metabolic:
- Hyper-/hypoglycaemia
- Hypercalcaemia

Iatrogenic:
- Medication-induced
- Toxins (organophosphates, arsenic)

Neoplastic:
- Intracranial mass
- Paraneoplastic syndromes
- Ovarian cyst rupture

Congenital:
- Epilepsy/seizures

Other:
- Migraines
- Pregnancy
- Bulimia nervosa
- Conversion disorder

Before starting

Establish rapport:
- Introduce yourself
- Obtain consent from the patient: "I'll be asking you questions, and then performing a physical examination to find out why you are vomiting. Is this OK with you?"
- Expose the patient: when the physical examination is required

Confirm patient details:
- Name   *Judith McNeil*
- Age   *35 years*
- Occupation   *Librarian*

History

History of presenting complaint
- History of vomiting: *started 1 day ago, worsening, worse with food, not bilious or faeculant*
- Associated symptoms:
  - Abdominal pain: *vague, dull pain that localises to suprapubic/right lower quadrant (RLQ)*
  - Constipation or diarrhoea: *no*
  - Headaches: *no*
  - Vertigo: *no*
  - Fevers/chills: *no*

- New medication: *no*
- Loss of weight / loss of appetite: *no*
- Last menstruation: *3/52 ago, periods usually regular monthly*
- Denies all else

Past medical history and family history

- *Endometriosis – had two previous laparoscopies*
- *Chronic back pain*
- *Mother had bowel cancer at age 45 years, father had heart problems*

Drug history and allergies

- *Celecoxib, pantoprazole*
- *NKDA*

Social history

- Smoking history: *non-smoker*
- Alcohol and drugs history: *social drinker, nil illicit drugs*
- *Lives at home with husband and two children*

Examination

General inspection (ABCD-V)

- **A**ppearance: *appears comfortable*
- **B**ody habitus: *overweight, BMI 26*
- **C**ognition: *patient is conscious and oriented*
- **D**evices / **D**rugs: *nil*

Investigations

BBMI-O: Bedside, **B**loods, **M**icrobiology, **I**maging and **O**ther

- **V**itals: *BP 120/75mmHg, HR 80bpm, RR 17 per minute; oxygen saturation at 100% on room air; temperature 37.2°C*

Neurological examination

- *Cranial nerves, upper and lower limbs all intact*
- *No hearing loss / nystagmus, Dix–Hallpike negative*

Gastrointestinal examination

- Inspection:
  - *No abdominal distension, multiple small scars from previous laparoscopy sites*
- Palpation:
  - *Mildly tender in RLQ*
  - *No peritonism*
  - *No cross tenderness / percussion tenderness*
  - *No hepatosplenomegaly*
  - *No inguinal / femoral hernias*
  - *Rovsing's sign negative*
- Percussion:
  - *No shifting dullness*
  - *No percussive tenderness*
- Auscultation:
  - *Bowel sounds present, high-pitched tinkling*

Renal examination

- *No flank tenderness*
- *No suprapubic tenderness*

Investigation	Rationale
Bedside	
Urine dipstick	Looking for signs of UTI
Bloods:	
FBC	Looking for raised WCC or low Hb
CRP	Looking for infection
U&Es and creatinine	Looking for renal impairment / electrolyte abnormality
CMP	Looking for electrolyte abnormality / hypercalcaemia
Coagulation studies	Looking for raised INR / preoperative planning
LFTs	Looking for acutely deranged liver function

Investigation	Rationale
Lipase	Looking for pancreatitis
BSL + ketones	Looking for hypo- / hyperglycaemia
Beta-hCG	Looking for raised beta-hCG in pregnancy
Microbiology	
Urine MCS	Looking for haematuria / bacteriuria
Imaging	
AXR	Investigate for air-fluid levels, volvulus
US abdomen	Investigate for ovarian pathology
CT abdomen / pelvis	Investigate for acute abdomen causes, transition point in acute obstruction
CT brain	Consider if investigating raised intracranial pressure
Other	
Vestibular function testing	Consider if investigating vertigo

Diagnosis

Small bowel obstruction secondary to intra-abdominal adhesions

Although appendicitis is also another important differential, given this patient is afebrile, does not have anorexia / nausea and examines relatively benignly, it is more likely her presentation is related to her previous abdominal procedures.

Management

Small bowel obstructions should be managed primarily by a surgical team. Definitive management is by exploratory laparotomy; however, select cases of non-complicated small bowel obstruction may be managed expectantly.

Initial management entails:
- Fluid resuscitation
- Strict nil by mouth
- Insertion of a nasogastric tube
- Obtaining of CT abdomen / pelvis to investigate for complications of small bowel obstruction

If symptoms improve or resolution of obstruction occurs, diet can be upgraded approximately every 24 hours in the following order:

- Clear fluids only
- Free fluids
- Light ward diet
- Full ward diet

Complications of small bowel obstruction indicating exploratory laparotomy include:
- Perforation
- Ischaemia demonstrated on CT
- Clinical deterioration or worsening of symptoms

Other differential diagnoses

- Appendicitis
- Abdominal migraine
- Food poisoning
- Viral gastroenteritis

Station 68 **Weight loss**

A 42-year-old man presents with a 3-month history of weight loss.

Tasks

1 Take a history
2 Perform physical examination

3 Provide rationale for investigations
4 Formulate a management plan

Differential diagnoses (VIITAMINC)

Vascular

Infective:
- Chronic infection (tuberculosis, HIV)

Inflammatory:
- Chronic obstructive pulmonary disease (COPD)
- Peptic ulcer disease
- Gastroparesis
- Inflammatory bowel disease
- Chronic pancreatitis

Trauma

Autoimmune

Metabolic:
- Hyperthyroidism

- Diabetes
- Phaeochromocytoma

Iatrogenic:
- Drug-induced (metformin, alcohol, amphetamines)

Neoplastic:
- Malignancy

Congenital:
- Coeliac disease

Other:
- Excessive exercise
- Eating disorder
- Depression
- Malnutrition

Before starting

Establish rapport:
- Introduce yourself
- Obtain consent from the patient: "I'll be asking you questions, and then performing a physical examination to find out why you are losing weight. Is this OK with you?"
- Expose the patient: when physical examination is required

Confirm patient details:
- Name — *Jason Webb*
- Age — *42 years*
- Occupation — *Construction worker*

History

History of presenting complaint

- History of weight loss: *gradual weight loss over the last 3 months, 10kg total, unintentional*
- Associated symptoms:
  - Change in appetite: *increased appetite*
  - Anxiety: *yes*
  - Tremor: *yes*
  - Palpitations: *yes*
  - Abdominal pain or nausea / vomiting: *no*
  - Diarrhoea: *no*
  - Fevers / chills / rigors: *no*
  - Cardiorespiratory symptoms: *no*
  - Lethargy: *no*

Past medical history and family history

- *Nil significant past medical history*
- *Mother had depression and COPD, father was an alcoholic*

Drug history and allergies

- *Nil*
- *NKDA*

Social history

- Smoking history: *non-smoker*
- Alcohol and drugs history: *social drinker, nil illicit drugs*
- *Lives at home with wife*

Examination

General inspection (ABCD-V)

- **A**ppearance: *healthy looking man, anxious and sweaty*
- **B**ody habitus: *BMI 24*
- **C**ognition: *Glasgow Coma Scale (GCS) 15*
- **D**evices / **D**rugs: *nil*
- **V**itals: *BP 130/80mmHg, HR 95bpm, RR 17 per minute; oxygen saturation at 100% on room air; temperature 36.8°C*

Gastrointestinal examination

- Inspection:
  - *No abdominal distension or scars indicating previous surgery*

- Palpation:
  - *Abdomen soft and non-tender*
  - *No hepatosplenomegaly*
  - *No masses palpable*
- Percussion:
  - *Resonant bowel, no percussion tenderness*
- Auscultation:
  - *Normal bowel sounds present*

Thyroid examination

- Inspection:
  - *Mild goitre present*
  - *Enhanced physiological tremor*
  - *Some proptosis of bilateral eyes, no ophthalmoplegia*
- Palpation:
  - *Palpable diffuse thyroid swelling in anterior neck*
  - *No nodules*
  - *No cervical lymphadenopathy*
- Percussion:
  - *No retrosternal expansion*
- Auscultation:
  - *No bruits heard over the thyroid gland*

Cardiorespiratory examination

- *Heart sounds dual with no murmurs*
- *Bilateral vesicular breath sounds*

Investigations

BBMI-O: Bedside, **B**loods, **M**icrobiology, **I**maging and **O**ther

Investigation	Rationale
Bedside	
Bloods	
FBC	Looking for raised WCC
ESR / CRP	Looking for inflammation
TFTs	Looking for hyperthyroidism
TSI, TRAbs, anti-TPO antibody	Looking for autoimmune thyroid diseases (Graves', Hashimoto's, etc.)
U&Es and creatinine	Looking for renal impairment / electrolyte abnormality
CMP	Looking for electrolyte abnormality

Investigation	Rationale
Lipase	Looking for pancreatitis
Blood sugar level	Looking for hypo-/hyperglycaemia
Albumin, folic acid, B$_{12}$, TTR	Looking for malnutrition
Anti-tTG, anti-DGP, HLA-DQ2, HLA-DQ8	Looking for coeliac disease
Microbiology	
QuantiFERON Gold	If considering tuberculosis
HIV assay	If considering HIV
Imaging	
US neck ± FNA	Investigate for thyroid mass
CT abdomen/pelvis	Investigate for chronic gastrointestinal pathology
CT neck	Consider if investigating thyroid mass
Thyroid scan	Assess for cause of hyperthyroidism
Other	
Gastroscopy/colonoscopy	Consider if investigating gastrointestinal disorders
Faecal elastase, faecal fat	Consider if investigating chronic pancreatitis
Echocardiography	Consider if investigating for cardiorespiratory disease
Pulmonary function tests	Consider if investigating for cardiorespiratory disease

Diagnosis

Graves' disease

A patient with known family history of thyroid disease that presents with hyperthyroidism and a goitre must be investigated thoroughly for Graves'.

The gold standard investigation to confirm Graves' disease is TSH receptor antibody (TRAb).

Management

Treatment of Graves' disease revolves around management of hyperthyroidism and management of ophthalmopathy.

Management of hyperthyroidism

- Medical:
  - Antithyroid medications are given to reduce thyroid hormone levels (carbimazole, propylthiouracil)
  - Radioactive iodine can be used if patients do not respond to antithyroid medications

■ Surgical:
  ● Hemi- or total thyroidectomy is a last resort consideration

Management of ophthalmopathy

■ Medical:
  ● Local treatments (eye lubricants, taping of eyes at night) are good for mild disease
  ● Severe disease may require glucocorticoids or orbital decompression

Other differential diagnoses

■ Diabetes
■ Inflammatory bowel disease
■ Coeliac disease
■ Chronic pancreatitis
■ Malignancy
■ Eating disorder
■ Depression

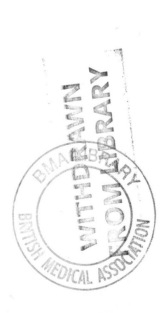